Praise for *Parenting at Your Child's P*

"With humility, warmth, and good humor, Dr. Gator sh
he's gained as a holistically inspired pediatrician and
parent. *Parenting at Your Child's Pace* is a therapeutic, caln
bath, parents will feel their anxiety evaporating from the very first page."

—Janet Lansbury, bestselling author of
No Bad Kids and *Elevating Child Care*

"This book is a godsend for navigating all the challenges of being a new parent. Dr. Gator has become a go-to resource for raising healthy and happy kids in our modern-day world."

—Vani Hari, *New York Times* bestselling author and
founder of FoodBabe.com and Truvani

"For health-conscious parents who want to raise their children with the best of both Western medicine and complementary healing practices, this book is a must-read. Dr. Gator presents thoughtful, evidence-based information in his signature open-minded and inclusive style so that parents can make empowered and informed decisions. For the parents who say, 'I wish parenting came with an instruction manual,' your wish has been granted! Thank you, Dr. Gator, for putting kids first!"

—Dr. Ashley Mayer, aka Dr. Green Mom

"Having a pediatrician is a must, but having a pediatrician that listens, considers your family's needs, and supports well-rounded health is an incredible bonus. In this book, Dr. Joel takes you through the intricate, sometimes scary maze of raising your infant. From the initial moments your baby is put into your care, throughout the many months ahead, Dr. Joel helps you understand how your child is growing and guides you through it all with his knowledge. In times of questions and need, and all the in-betweens, you will find in Dr. Joel's book a wealth of information to support this incredible journey of your child's health as a whole."

—Dr. Siggie, PhD

"Dr. Joel Warsh, backed by extensive research and a compassionate approach, empowers parents with the knowledge to confidently navigate their children's unique development. He champions informed decision-making while reminding families that every child blossoms at their own pace."

—Tara Clark, creator of Modern Mom Probs

"Dr. Gator has been an incredibly supportive and respectful sounding board for our family. I'm so grateful for his integrative and evidence-based approach to caring for his patients, including our two children. Ages zero to three are transformative, for everyone. The more support, the better!"

—Daniella Monet Gardner, actress, singer, and wellness entrepreneur

"Dr. Warsh has been a calm voice of reason in the midst of the chaos and polarizing views that come along with being a first-time parent. He provides a necessary balance of holistic, preventative health while continuing to utilize the advantages of modern medicine when appropriate. This book has a wealth of information that will educate parents without overwhelming them, as Dr. Warsh takes a warm but no-nonsense approach."

—Ashley Greene (Khoury), actress

"There's never been a more pressing time for parents to be in the driver's seat of their child's health. Dr. Gator and *Parenting at Your Child's Pace* transforms parents' anxiety to confidence and empowerment so they can worry less and enjoy more of their child's first three years of life."

—Dr. Elana Roumell, founder of Med School for Moms

"Dr. Gator is facilitating conversation in spaces where it is taboo to ask questions. This is incredibly important for parents looking for truly health-conscious and inclusive care for their children. Instead of leaning into the unnecessary and unhelpful pressures of being 'politically correct,' Dr. Gator's approach creates real conversations that serve to strengthen Western medicine as the modern savior that it is, but also make space for generations of wisdom that holistic medicine provides in preventative spaces. This book brings together both disciplines in a balanced and complementary way that gives parents the tools they need to make the best possible decisions for their family's health."

—Natalia Rodriguez, founder of Create Kids

"A much-needed book that will change the way you think about your child's health and well-being with evidence-backed pathways to empower you to make confident and informed decisions to promote their lifelong well-being."

—Shikha Gill, founder of My Little Food Critic

Parenting at Your Child's Pace

Parenting at Your Child's Pace

THE INTEGRATIVE PEDIATRICIAN'S GUIDE TO THE FIRST THREE YEARS

JOEL WARSH, MD, MSc

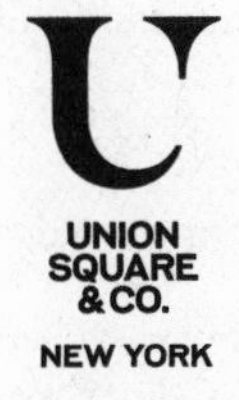

UNION SQUARE & CO.
NEW YORK

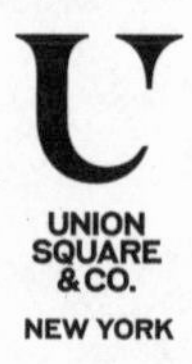

UNION SQUARE & CO. and the distinctive Union Square & Co. logo are trademarks of Sterling Publishing Co., Inc.

Union Square & Co., LLC, is a subsidiary of Sterling Publishing Co., Inc.

This publication is intended for informational purposes only. The publisher does not claim that this publication shall provide or guarantee any benefits, healing, cure, or any results in any respect. This publication is not intended to provide or replace medical advice, treatment, or diagnosis or be a substitute to consulting with a physician or other licensed medical or health-care providers. The publisher and author shall not be liable or responsible for any use or application of any content contained in this publication or any adverse effects, consequence, loss, or damage of any type resulting or arising from, directly or indirectly, the use or application of any content contained in this publication.

The author and editor have made every effort to reproduce the substance of the conversations relied on in this book but some have been edited and condensed for clarity and space. Names and identifying details have been changed at the individuals' request and/or to preserve the author's obligation to uphold patient confidentiality.

ISBN 978-1-4549-5249-7
ISBN 978-1-4549-5250-3 (e-book)

Library of Congress Control Number: 2024003581
Library of Congress Cataloging-in-Publication Data is available upon request.

For information about custom editions, special sales, and premium purchases, please contact specialsales@unionsquareandco.com.

Printed in Canada

2 4 6 8 10 9 7 5 3 1

unionsquareandco.com

Cover design by Sara Wood
Cover image by bsd studio/iStock/Getty Images Plus
Interior design by Rich Hazelton

To my incredible wife, Sarah Intelligator, the woman behind the name Dr. Gator, and to my family and friends. This book is a testament to the love, guidance, and strength you've all provided. It's because of each of you that these pages are filled with the wisdom I hope to share. Thank you.

CONTENTS

INTRODUCTION

A few months into opening my pediatric clinic, Integrative Pediatrics, the client base started to shift. Initially, my patient pool consisted mostly of families from my old practice who already favored the integrative approach—often labeled as "crunchy." Then, randomly (or so I thought), celebrities and other industry bigwigs started bringing their children to see me. More exciting to me, though, were the decidedly non-crunchy families from across Los Angeles, from diverse backgrounds, that began coming as well. I know I'm really dating myself when I say I truly felt like Kevin Costner's character in *Field of Dreams*: "If you build it, they will come." I discovered that many of these families, including my celebrity patients, learned of my office through word of mouth—chatting with other parents at preschool drop-off, Saturday soccer meets, dance recitals, and PTA fundraisers.

These were (and are) parents who, at their core, respect and believe in modern medicine, but felt disempowered by the limitations of how it tends to be practiced. They felt unheard (and even dismissed) when they broached topics beyond the realm of acute treatment. These were parents who said YES to Western medicine, but NO to over-prescription and aggressive treatment, YES to complementary therapies and preventive choices, but NO to woo-woo practitioners and out-there claims. They were interested in organic food, toxin-free homes, and the ways diet and lifestyle can lay the foundation for their child's lifelong health. They Botoxed *and* breastfed (and wanted to know if it's safe to do both simultaneously). They were families with a mom and a dad, two dads, two moms, single parents, adoptive parents, and every other configuration you can imagine—from all walks of life—seeking care that embodied their values: care that embraces body, mind, and spirit and is open-minded, balanced, truly health-conscious, holistic, and inclusive. Sound like you? Welcome.

As a board-certified, practicing pediatrician with a master's degree in epidemiology and community health, who happens to go by the nickname "Dr. Gator" (it's not a Florida thing; it grew out of my wife's last name, Intelligator), I work with and talk to parents and children every single day, integrating complementary healing practices with my training in traditional Western medicine. While I believe in the incredible power of Western medicine—much of which I would describe as nothing short of miraculous—I don't think it's sacrilegious to ask questions about how we employ it and to seek additional tools for our healing and wellness arsenals. I bridge the unnecessary and unhelpful divide between nature-made and lab-made, alternative and conventional, East and West. Just as I integrate complementary practices with my training in traditional Western medicine, I also feel strongly that parents should be empowered to integrate different parenting philosophies and techniques that work for them—rather than feeling pressured to be a strict adherent of one method or another.

When my patients come to me with a question, be it about medications, supplements, toileting, or time-outs, my goal is to provide context, debunk misinformation, and help them synthesize good information so that they can make confident, empowered choices. That may mean combining techniques or sticking with the tried and true. In the end, my goal is to unite the divide between "the right way" and the way that is right for *your* child. My patients don't have to choose a side—just do what makes sense for their family, within the bounds of "reasonable and safe." It's what I like to call "parenting at your child's pace."

You won't find any proselytizing or preaching here. You *will* find a thoughtful synthesis, evidence-backed options, and critical thinking strategies to help modern parents like you determine a path forward based on informed decision making that works for your child. *Parenting at Your Child's Pace* is a guide to thinking through the health concerns and developmental changes that come up during the first three years of life so that you, the parent, are equipped with the information to make confident choices, while navigating the unique realities of parenting today.

The SEEDS of Well-Being

Ultimately, when I work with families, my goal—beyond doing everything I can to help secure the well-being of your children, of course—is to bridge the divide between doctor and patient (or the patient's caregiver, as is the case in pediatrics). I want parents to trust their judgment, feel confident in their choices, and be empowered to implement both integrative health and integrative parenting practices at home. After all, I became a pediatrician to help kids—and the well-being of kids starts at home.

Since I run a private practice, I am fortunate to have more time than most doctors with each of my patients. For me this means more listening and less talking, more teaching and less telling. It means seeing each child as a unique individual and learning all the factors that may impact their health. It means taking the time to understand the specific needs of each family too.

The reality is that children's health and parenting often lack one-size-fits-all solutions. Yet many parents don't feel confident making choices tailored to their own children's needs. It doesn't help that most health and wellness advice out there seems to promote its own "Magic Smoothie" recipe that "cures all"—literally and figuratively. Few things make me angrier than the perpetuation of these kinds of fairy tales: There is no one-size-fits-all plan when it comes to health. There is no diet that will work for everyone. Nor is there one way to live or one way to eat. But there are many lifestyle choices you can make to optimize your child's resilience and bolster his or her future health. Making the right choices is predicated on our understanding the five factors that have the greatest impact on our physical, mental, and emotional health. I call these factors the SEEDS of well-being: Stress, Environment, Exercise, Diet, and Sleep.

Stress: Children, although resilient, are not impervious to the weight of stress, be it stress in the home due to marriage and family dynamics, or the stress of life transitions, and so on.

Environment: Equally significant is the environment they inhabit. A child's developing system is more sensitive to toxins found in their surroundings, from the air they breathe to the very products that touch their skin. The importance of wholesome interaction with nature, through clean air and toxin-free spaces, cannot be overstated.

Exercise: Physical activity, too, holds a prominent role in a child's health, extending beyond mere physical development. It lays the groundwork for mental agility, resilience, and an enduring appreciation for movement. For young children, this can be as simple as going for walks with them or adding more tummy time.

Diet: Coupled with the above is the pivotal role of diet. The foods that children consume are the building blocks of their present and future health, shaping everything from cognitive capabilities to emotional stability.

Sleep: Last, but by no means least, is the transformative power of sleep. Often sidelined in discussions, quality sleep acts as the cornerstone for emotional regulation, memory consolidation, and overall rejuvenation. It's during these restful hours that the young body repairs and grows, setting the stage for a new day filled with endless possibilities.

By recognizing and integrating the SEEDS of well-being into our children's lives from their first day of life, we offer them more than immediate remedies; we gift them a foundation of lifelong wellness rooted in nature's wisdom. In a medical system that tends to focus somewhat narrowly on treatment, prevention too often takes a backseat. Don't get me wrong, if you have a bad case of pneumonia, I'm damn thankful (as I am certain are you) that lifesaving antibiotics exist. But acute disease is not the only problem we're dealing with these days in medicine. Just as big an issue, if not bigger, is chronic disease. More than half of Americans and nearly half of all children now have a chronic disease—something that was not the case fifty years ago, or even ten years ago. However, when parents focus on the SEEDS of well-being they take back their power to alter the current trajectory of chronic disease. The poor sleep, unhealthy diets, and toxin-filled homes of today are the future chronic conditions of tomorrow.

No, this is not merely my opinion (though just wait, you are about to hear my opinion aplenty). Countless studies have shown that lifestyle changes can and do lead to better overall health outcomes. And while I stand by my rule that if you encounter a health-care, wellness, or fitness guru (or any guru, really) who comes onto social media or the latest talk show touting their magical smoothie, you should run the other way, I do have my own recipe for integrative parenting to offer you. No, the Dr. Gator smoothie isn't a literal blend of fruits and vegetables. Instead, it starts with a large scoop of SEEDS, to which I add a generous dollop of the essential elements needed for a balanced, holistic approach to your child's well-being. It's about nurturing not just your child's physical health but also his or her mental, emotional, and social wellness, because in the end we cannot separate health—and preventing chronic disease—from our children's overall well-being in body, mind, and spirit.

The Pediatrician's Perspective: Navigating Parenthood Beyond the Medical Advice

When my wife was pregnant with our son, people would often joke about how nice it must be to be a pediatrician (or married to one)—implying that I knew all there was to know when it came to babies. The truth is, I was scared and nervous. Being a pediatrician doesn't *really* prepare you to be a parent; it prepares you to deal with health complications. By the time my son arrived, I was able to identify whether or not his late-night crying and tugging at his ear indicated a likely ear infection or just plain old newborn fussiness. I felt confident that I knew the difference between a normal-looking poop and one that should be investigated further. I had a pretty good sense of normal spit-up versus reflux disease. Yet I was no professional when it came to rocking my newborn to sleep. Helping my wife navigate painful breastfeeding and mastitis was new to me. I had never before swaddled a baby.

My point? Even professional child specialists start off parenthood experiencing impostor syndrome. Take this baby home? *Me?* There is certainly some advantage to being a physician . . . but, in all honesty, not in a significant way. If anything, sometimes doctors are *more* nervous about everything—we know all about the bad and rare stuff. Doctors also struggle with information overload, and I can promise you that medical credentials do not obviate those frantic Google searches. The internet is a firehose of competing advice—from social media to podcasts to simple web searches—that inevitably seems to imply imminent disaster at every turn. Every click leads to another opinion, rendering trustworthy answers prized, albeit elusive, gems.

And don't forget that along with both good and bad information on the internet, there are also countless books, cultural truisms, and the often-perplexing "wisdom" of our own parents—who were raised by people with decidedly different generational values and had children in a time quite different from our own.

The new parents I work with tend to fall into two groups when it comes to the results of their scrolling habits: either they think the newborn period is supposed to be a perfect and magical time of snuggling, inhaling that new baby smell, and taking picturesque walks with their perfectly wrapped potato (and camera crew with full lighting and sound in tow), or they're frantic inhalers of statistics, worst-case scenarios, best practices, and articles on exactly how many pees a newborn needs to have on day three of life or when exactly to introduce potential allergens to best prevent the possibility of a food allergy. The first group inevitably feels confused and betrayed by reality and, worse, ashamed that they must be doing things wrong (otherwise, why would it be so hard?). The latter group inevitably feels woefully unprepared the more they read. So, of course, they keep reading. They have thirty different half-read parenting books on their coffee table—some of which spout conflicting advice, further engendering a bevy of anxieties. And the first group almost always become members of the second group.

One patient's mom, Amelia, particularly illustrated this point for me. I first met her when she was pregnant with my soon-to-be patient. She came in for a prenatal interview, which is usually the time when parents assess whether or not my practice is a good fit for their family. I expected

THE DR. GATOR SMOOTHIE

Introducing the Dr. Gator Smoothie—a guide to holistic parenting. Although research supports the benefits of a holistic approach to pediatric care for improving overall health outcomes, I want to clarify something important: if you ever come across any self-proclaimed "guru" promising miraculous results through a single smoothie, be skeptical. That being said, what I offer you with the Dr. Gator Smoothie is not a miracle cure, but a carefully crafted recipe designed to complement a balanced, integrative approach to your family's health and wellness.

1. **Emotionally Nurturing Spaces: Craft home environments that keep your kids not only safe but also emotionally enriched. Spend time in nature.**
2. **Mental Health Support: Your mental health, as well as that of your child, is one of the most important factors that will lead to an overall healthy child.**
3. **Mindful Stress Management and Resilience: Managing your stress effectively not only supports your mental health but also sets a positive example for your little one.**
4. **Social Support: Encouraging friendships and social interactions and maintaining your own will improve your child's emotional well-being and communication skills.**
5. **Regular Physical Activity: Encouraging regular exercise supports physical development and can instill a lifelong love of physical activity.**

6. **Adequate Sleep: Ensuring you and your children get enough sleep is vital for their growth and cognitive development.**
7. **Balanced Nutrition: Consume a variety of foods, including fresh, local, organic fruits and vegetables, and healthy proteins and fats, while limiting sugar, processed foods, and anything premade or prepackaged. Prepare foods at home. Make your baby foods where you can. Cooking more is one of the most important things you can do to build a healthy family.**
8. **Limiting Toxins: Reduce exposure to harmful substances such as dyes, preservatives, pesticides, and plastics. Read the labels on everything you buy. Learn to be a proactive consumer.**
9. **Access to Health Care: Regular checkups ensure that your child's health is continually monitored and protected.**
10. **Limited Tobacco Exposure: Keep your child's environment free from smoke.**
11. **Clean Air and Water: Ensuring access to clean air and water is critical for overall health.**
12. **Strong Community Ties: A supportive community can foster a sense of belonging and security.**
13. **Love and Affection: Shower your child with love and affection. This emotional nourishment is just as important as physical nutrition.**

her to quiz me about my approach to medicine, interventions, and office policies. Instead, with stars in her eyes, she spent approximately fifteen minutes describing her ideal nursery, detailing a Pinterest-perfect picture of idyllic motherhood moments. As she ran through a checklist of baby, and even toddler, products recommended by her mom friends, she wanted to know whether I thought she should buy them too.

Listening to Amelia, I felt a sinking feeling in my gut. I knew she was in for a gargantuan reality check. She was worried about the wrong things. I tried my best to gently steer the conversation toward more useful topics, like what happens during a well visit, and away from toddler toys. I opined that I didn't think any of the products she mentioned would significantly improve her or her baby's quality of life in the newborn months.

After her baby, Max, was born, Amelia really began to struggle. Max was colicky. Amelia felt overwhelmed, defeated by the realities of a hard-to-soothe baby and the endless sleepless nights. She turned to the internet for solace and became a voracious consumer of any and all parenting advice, especially concerning the "causes" of colic. She was convinced there was something wrong with Max. On top of that, she developed a fixation on his totally normal and, frankly, very minor baby acne, admitting to me at his one-month checkup that she felt embarrassed about it: "I can't get a perfect one-month photo," she whispered, as she shared with me that she had been documenting each week's anniversary of his birth online. To me, Max was perfect: he was gaining weight appropriately, was meeting all of his "milestones," and was one of the cutest newborns to cross the threshold of my office that week.

In time, with some guidance and support, Amelia learned to trust her instincts as a mother, finding a balance between seeking advice and valuing her own intuition. She also learned to shut off her phone when she was getting stressed. During one visit, her eyes welled up with tears as she confided in me. "I thought I was failing because the reality of life with Max wasn't picture-perfect. Then I feared I was failing because I couldn't keep up with all the advice out there, or it didn't seem to make a difference when I did." It was a humbling reminder for me that in the midst of our digital age, personal, tailored advice and understanding can make a world of difference—not to mention simply putting down the phone.

People! We are currently living in the most technologically advanced age humans have ever known. At the pace that technology is advancing, you may be reading this book on Mars or downloading it to your brain (scary thought, I know). When it comes to birth and newborns, we are living in a very low risk moment in history, with the most support and expertise anyone has ever had at our fingertips. Take a step back from the hustle and bustle of modern life and think back to just a few decades ago.

For example, radium was hailed as a miracle substance and found its way into everyday items like toothpaste and food, only for us to later discover its radioactive dangers. Fortunately or unfortunately (depending on which way you look at it), our children are now way less likely to end up a comic book superhero. Similarly, parents used to administer morphine to infants to help them sleep, unaware of its addictive nature and the serious respiratory issues it could cause. Those babies probably slept really well, though. Until the 1970s, the widespread use of leaded gasoline and paint exposed children to a toxic substance now known to lower IQ and cause serious health complications, especially in babies who often chewed on painted toys or ingested paint chips.

Even though no one was able to pull up a list of Oprah's favorite nursery items five hundred years ago (or even as recently as thirty years ago), I promise you that new parents still lived to tell the tale. They survived and thrived. And when they didn't, it wasn't because of a lack of wipe warmers or white noise machines; it was because childbirth was incredibly dangerous and the infectious diseases that killed infants and young children had ineffective treatments—or none at all. Trust me, we are doing fine.

The mere fact that you are reading this book means you are already starting from a place of major okayness—you're not in the middle of traveling across the Oregon Trail or fleeing a war-torn region. You're literate, you have some leisure time, and you care. We have so much our ancestors never had, and most people still managed to raise healthy and well-adjusted children. Prior generations did not have the internet at their fingertips and had to navigate the Dewey decimal system, track down a textbook, and read it. This wasn't that long ago. If anything, we now have too much information. So, consider this your official permission to step away from Google. It's great to be informed, but I came away from medical school with an understanding that the information never ends. You can study forever and still feel unprepared for the exam. Endless scrolling won't make you better at parenting (and it might just make things worse). Every child is unique, and the challenges will vary from child to child, parent to parent. You will figure it out as you go. I promise.

Sometimes you will need to learn something new. When you're frantically combing the internet for information, I caution you to be extremely wary of anyone who claims to have all the answers—especially when they don't know your child. Hell, I definitely don't have all the answers. I do promise you, though, I'll help you navigate everything from those high-anxiety newborn months to the throes of toddlerhood and arrive at answers that make sense for your family. Rather than tell you what to do or how to do it, I'm going to equip you with tools, share ways to think through risks and benefits, and ultimately dispense with the bullshit, so that you feel confident and empowered to make the best choices for *your* child.

You Got This

As a doctor in Los Angeles, I work with families from a spectrum of backgrounds, including some with significant means and lots of help. But even those LA producer/agent power couples with the night nurse ask the same questions and share the same anxieties. When they are first-time parents, almost nobody thinks "I got this!" Nobody feels ready. I don't care how much money you have, or how big a celebrity you are, the questions—and the fear—remain the same. At the end of the day, money cannot buy most of the things that you *really* need in the first few weeks and months with your baby. No matter your socioeconomic class, career, ethnicity, religion, or gender, parenthood leaves virtually every human being on equal footing. The recipe for parenthood in those early days is: a heap of love, a sprinkle of patience, a dash of bravery, a pinch of humility, a generous helping of a tolerance for bodily fluids that are not your own, and *sleep (when you can get it)*.

In some ways, the problem is *how much* some of us do have. It's hard not to feel unprepared when multiple industries exist to make you feel that way, so that you'll click through that influencer's links and add to cart. Tomorrow, a friendly delivery person will magically drop off whatever you ordered (encased in way too much cardboard and plastic). All too soon, your home will grow into a jungle of gadgets, gizmos, and gear, each of which promises to be the ultimate solution to your parenting woes. Amid this barrage of items, the irony emerges: all of these things you don't need—deceptively masquerading themselves as "essentials"—are precisely what are stressing you out. The clutter becomes both a physical and mental obstacle, obscuring the simple joys of parenting. You can't buy your way to being a good parent and, more important, you don't need to. The essence of good parenting lies in care and connection. As parents, our undivided attention and unwavering love outweigh any material possession we can offer. Even a diaper change is an opportunity to give your child the attention he or she needs. Simply put, great parenting is about being present and caring.

There are few things scarier than becoming a parent for the first time (except, maybe, the moment you realize they expect you to take the baby home). You feel you have no idea what you're doing. *Everyone* feels that way. Because nobody who hasn't had a kid has had a kid. Now, while double negatives are always a fun brainteaser, I'm telling you this so that you *stop*, right now, comparing yourself to other parents. Yes, we all arrive at parenthood with different resources (emotional, psychological, social, financial, cultural). *But* we also start at the same place: a place that, alongside the joy, is filled with uncertainty. We worry that we're not good enough, that we won't do a good job, that we don't know how, that we are going to . . . well, fuck it up.

When my wife, Sarah, read the initial draft of this book, and, in particular, the newborn section, she joked, "I thought the point of this book was to make parents feel *less* stressed, but some of these topics, like sudden infant death syndrome, are pretty terrifying." Ironically, her sentiment runs contrary to the book's intent. Although some topics are inherently stressful, as a physician I am obligated to inform you of the *worst*-case scenario—those situations that occur with less frequent regularity but are nonetheless *possible*. I would be irresponsible if I did not attune you to the issues that should be cause for genuine concern; I would be remiss if I did not share with you the common questions I am asked and the issues I encounter on a daily basis in my pediatric practice. After all, this information is integral to your treasure trove of parenting knowledge. However, the true purpose of this book is threefold:

1. To warn you of the *possible* and the *likely*, while arming you with the information and confidence necessary to navigate *both*.

2. To *decrease* the stress and pressures associated with parenting, often imposed by social media influencers, internet forums, other parents, well-intentioned family members, and, yes, even the medical profession itself.

3. To empower *you* to make decisions that are right for *you* and *your child* (irrespective of all the noise) because parenting is not a one-size-fits-all proposition.

My sincere hope is that, after reading this book, you walk away feeling a little less pressure to conform to the picture-perfect parenting *fantasy* promulgated by your social media feed, pause before judging your child or parenting based on arbitrary factors, and use the information gleaned from these pages—coupled with your innate and trustworthy parental intuition—to confidently make decisions without second-guessing yourself at every turn. Buddha is quoted as having said, "Happiness is a journey, not a destination." When we get so caught up in the unattainable quest for a subjective construct, such as perfection, we deprive ourselves of the daily joys along the way. Although at times, parenting demands so much of us, ultimately, it *is* a joy—one of the greatest in life!

In the 1940s, in his groundbreaking first book, *Baby and Child Care,* Dr. Benjamin Spock promised mothers, "you know more than you think you do," encouraging them to trust in themselves. It was and arguably remains a radical, albeit powerful, message. Dr. Spock's words still ring true today. The potential for extraordinary parenting is woven into your DNA.

My wish for you, dear reader, is that this book will leave you feeling like the parenting superhero you always were but simply never realized. View this book (yes, even that intimidating newborn section) as a tool of empowerment, rather than a catalyst for dejection. This book is aptly titled *Parenting at Your Child's Pace*. You have the esteemed honor and privilege to parent your child. You are not being asked to parent any other, so there is no need to look to other children or parents as a benchmark. At the risk of sounding cliché, children grow up so quickly. Enjoy the journey.

You got this.

SECTION I

Arrival

It's amazing how much can change in just one generation. I was born in the early '80s in Toronto, Canada. I have noticed that Americans tend to think of Canada as much more socially progressive than the US, at least when it comes to medical care (with our publicly funded, universal health care system and all). But Mount Sinai Hospital—the teaching hospital where I was born—and my mom's OB, Dr. Bernstein, were about as traditional as it came. The art and science of labor and delivery were not so different from what they were in the States at that time: lots of drugs offered, and lots of formula provided. Back then, the common wisdom was not to eat once labor started. As a result, when my mom went into the hospital on day three of labor, she was starving and was immediately administered IV fluids and an epidural upon her admittance. The doctor wanted her to sleep so she would be "rested" for the pushing; he was concerned she wouldn't have the strength otherwise because she hadn't eaten. (Am I the only one who sees the irony here?) My dad was allowed in the room while my mom gave birth, but it wasn't the coziest, most supportive environment. My mom still recalls the faceless heads (med students) staring at her through the observation window and a nurse jokingly remarking to my father "your wife's crotch is open prey to anybody now." As my head emerged, Dr. Bernstein commented I was "too pretty to be a boy." (This was before parents generally learned a baby's sex in utero.) My mom somewhat sarcastically responded, "Well, the decisive part is still to come." Ah, the '80s.

Nurses cleaned me, swaddled me, and whisked me away for checking immediately after I was born; my mom didn't get to hold me for another half hour. To say breastfeeding was not encouraged would be an understatement. By the time my sister was born a few years later, my mom remembers a greater push for breastfeeding. When I was born, bottle feeding was thought to be easier and formula was readily available and free in the hospital. Moms were encouraged to rest, sleep, and let the nurses handle things like feeding. I spent my first night of life in the nursery. Babies were taken to the nursery often; my mom estimates I was in the nursery (as opposed to in her room) for approximately half the time I was in the hospital. And from the time of my birth, how long was I in the hospital? Five days. Yep, you read that correctly. No, my mom did not have any postpartum issues and the birth itself was uncomplicated. That was just the way it was at the time. During the day, nurses gave my mom lessons on feeding, bathing, diapering, what have you. The environment was very hands-on and helpful. By the time my sister arrived three years later, the standard stay had shortened to two to three days. When my brother was born two years after that, they got the boot after just a day.

In some regards, change couldn't come quickly enough (separating a newborn from its mother?!). The hospital environment I was born into looks very alien today, whether you're in Canada, the United States, or anywhere else on planet Earth. When my own son, Eli, was born in Los Angeles, well into the twenty-first century, he got to snuggle on my wife's chest for as long as they both wanted, and Sarah's desire to begin breastfeeding right away was supported by the nurses and her OB/GYN, and was in alignment with the hospital mission. Other choices they were less simpatico with—for whatever reason, our preference to use the diapers and wipes we had brought with us, rather than the chemical-filled, hospital-provided wipes and diapers, was met with major attitude. (I promise we were neither self-righteous or holier-than-thou about this.) Heck, they were upset Sarah didn't want to take pain meds or a stool softener. When they offered her some anti-inflammatory meds to address post-birth swelling, Sarah replied, "What do you expect? I just pushed a baby out of there. No thank you."The nurse was insistent. So was Sarah. Sarah of course won that battle, but not before receiving a caustic evil eye from the nurse.

Let's be clear. I have spent a lot of time in the hospital, and I love the hospital nursery staff. They are generally the kindest people in the world. Still, labor and delivery through postpartum can be an arduous, exhausting, and emotional time. Sometimes your personal predilections don't quite align with the hospital's algorithm for care. Trust me, after you have a baby, you'll see what I mean. Always be kind to the staff, though. Even if you don't agree with everything. Just politely decline. They are there to keep you and your baby safe and healthy. You are on the same team. Don't forget that. But also don't think you won't be super annoyed at the littlest disturbances when you are exhausted. "We don't need anything, we're good" should suffice.

Finally, after about twenty-four hours, we were released, though to Sarah it felt like a million years. From the painful IV in her arm to the incessant blood pressure checks and tireless urging to take various medications, she was going crazy—not to mention from the mild power struggles with the less natural-minded nurses. Personally, I was very relieved to be going home, though more scared than I would've liked to admit. As a dad, in the hospital, I felt like there wasn't much I could really do. I tried to be helpful, but there was one little bed in our tiny room and I wasn't really doing a lot more than just being there, following the baby around, making sure that he was doing okay, and trying to support my wife. I felt kind of like a very exhausted cheerleader. I simultaneously felt a bit guilty that I was exhausted. Heck, I didn't really do any of the work. In the absence of anything to do, my mind was racing nonstop, thinking, when are we going to go home? What are we going to do next? Do we have all the stuff ready? Are we going to be able to get him to feed? I felt helpless.

Once your own bundle of joy arrives, whether you're the birthing parent or the support partner, you'll probably feel equal parts bliss and shell shock. The reality of those hours after birth may not be exactly what you imagined. You are exhausted, you haven't slept in a day. If you've just given birth, an entire staff of practitioners has seen every part of you. They unrelentingly poke and prod you. You feel less like a human being and more like a lab specimen. And now you have to recover while attempting to take care of a hungry, crying, and helpless new life that is entirely dependent on you.

For an uncomplicated vaginal birth, you can expect to be at the hospital for about a day or two after birth; for a non-emergency cesarean birth, you'll be there about three days. In this section, we'll cover what you can expect during a standard postpartum hospital stay, from the moments right after birth to the various procedures and interventions to which you'll need to consent or decline, to the typical concerns that might arise, and, finally, what you'll need to have sorted before they'll let you leave (hint: it's a car seat . . . and it's much less straightforward than it sounds). We'll cover the whats, the whys, and the hows, with the goal of arming you with the just right amount of information you need to make the right decisions for you, your child, and your family. The last thing you need when you're physically and emotionally depleted, running on adrenaline, and suddenly tasked with caring for your baby's life is to deal with decision fatigue. There are a bevy of universal aspects to having a newborn, including hospital procedures, sleepless nights, and managing visitors (though the approaches to handling each may vary). Meanwhile, newborn babies are accompanied by a number of strange and foreign issues. Learning how common some of these issues are will obviate that middle-of-the-night internet search rabbit hole, which always leads parents to dread the one-in-a-million worst-case scenario. While I can't completely rid you of the fear, anxiety, or feeling of helplessness, I do promise to assuage these feelings by demystifying this unknown terrain, rendering it easier to navigate. Welcome to parenthood.

The Moments After Birth

SKIN-TO-SKIN CONTACT

When it comes to skin-to-skin contact (SSC), if you are able, plan on it and do it, regardless of whether or not it's routine at your hospital or birth center (though, in the case of the latter, it's almost guaranteed to be standard operating procedure). What is skin-to-skin contact? It's exactly what it sounds like: immediately after birth (assuming the birth is full term and uncomplicated) or as soon as is possible, a newborn baby is placed, naked, belly down, on the bare chest of mom—hence, skin to skin. And yes, the baby is still covered in all of that birthing goo. At that point, baby is covered with a blanket for warmth, and mom and baby snuggle and bond as baby's reflexes and instincts kick in—wriggling toward and rooting for the breast for the first feed.

Back in the day, a nurse might have sponge-bathed a newborn before handing it over to the new parents, but the rise in practicing SSC following birth means immediate newborn bathing has largely fallen by the wayside. And delaying that first bath has a lot of other benefits too. Today, the World Health Organization (WHO) recommends holding off on bathing a newborn for twenty-four hours (or at least six hours if twenty-four isn't feasible). Why? Besides promoting bonding and breastfeeding (via SSC), waiting to bathe baby can help prevent drops in body temperature and blood sugar, while preserving the vernix (the waxy white coating covering newborn skin or, as I so eloquently referred to it earlier, the "goo"), which is naturally moisturizing and antibacterial, helping to protect delicate newborn skin. To some, this may be a little gross, or even like something out of the movie *Alien*. Yet there is no actual need to bathe your baby at the hospital (though if the nurse offers to teach you how to do it, and it's been more than twenty-four hours, there is no harm in learning that skill . . . especially if it'll lower your anxiety when it comes time to do it at home).

While I absolutely encourage breastfeeding (see page 123), I acknowledge that not all parents may be able to or want to. Regardless, the benefits of immediate to early SSC are so great for parent and baby, that it's worth doing no matter how you plan to feed your baby. It's one of the few newborn practices that has been widely studied and the results are as close to conclusive as it gets: skin-to-skin is awesome (that's the scientific term) for all involved.

Among the many benefits of SSC:

- Reduced maternal stress
- Easier delivery of the placenta
- Reduced maternal bleeding
- Releases oxytocin in birth parent that promotes bonding
- Familiarizes baby with birth parent's scent and voice, promoting bonding

- Helps establish breastfeeding
- Calms and relaxes both birth parent and baby (lowers heart rate and stress hormones)
- Stabilizes baby's heart rate and breathing
- Aids in regulating baby's body temperature
- May act as a prophylactic against postpartum depression and anxiety
- Enables transfer of friendly bacteria from birth parent's skin to baby's skin, protecting against infection

Of course, things don't always go as planned, and you may not be able to hold your baby immediately after birth. As hard as that is, know that researchers consider there to be three windows of initial SSC: immediate (immediately after birth), very early (thirty to forty minutes post-birth), and early (anytime in the twenty-four hours post-birth) in which many of the initial benefits of SSC, both to baby and parent, remain active.

There are no hard-and-fast rules concerning the duration of SSC, but the general guidelines suggest maintaining it until at least that first feeding or for an hour minimum, if possible. (Of course, hold your baby as long as you please—no one is saying you've got to let go after that first hour.)

Ultimately, there is no exact way SSC *has* to go. We want to foster attachment. We want mom to hold the baby, and we want to keep baby with mom as much as possible. We want to encourage breastfeeding if that's what mom wants to do, and, ideally, we don't want baby taken out of the room unless there is a health reason to do so. The more baby is on mom's chest, the better. SSC isn't something to worry about or try to get "right." If you've just given birth, you've already been through so much. In those first couple minutes of the baby's life, I wouldn't worry about anything other than placing your focus on and enjoying the baby, and keeping baby with you. If the baby is feeding, great. If baby falls asleep, great.

If your partner wants to hold baby, awesome. Partners can and should do SSC too. I held our little guy for the first time after about thirty minutes on mom. It was a bit weird at first (especially when he started angling for my nipple), but it was a perfect way to begin our bond. What's amazing about SSC is that its benefits extend beyond the mom. One study on fathers who practiced SSC after their infant's cesarean delivery showed that the fathers scored lower on markers of anxiety and depression than fathers who did not, as well as higher on indicators of "role attainment"—that is, identifying themselves as feeling like *active fathers.* I bring this up not only to encourage fathers, partners, and family to engage in SSC after the initial period with mom, but also because this study was done in the context of cesarean birth. More hospitals are encouraging immediate SSC after cesarean birth than used to do so. Surprisingly, it remains far less common than with vaginal birth—though there is no evidence to support avoiding it after a cesarean when mom is alert and up for it. Know this going in and don't be afraid to ask to hold your baby after a c-section. Don't be afraid to advocate for yourself—and your baby. After all, in a very real sense, SSC is a triumph in the ongoing effort to make medicine more humane and make birth itself less medicalized.

Before the twentieth century, mothers and newborns were rarely separated after birth. In the early 1900s, when birth started moving from the home to the hospital, things began to change. By the 1950s, women in the United States were giving birth almost exclusively in hospitals—and receiving pain relief for labor that made it difficult for them to care for their babies in the minutes and hours after delivery. This same pain relief often caused complications for babies—slow respiration, sluggishness, lower body temperatures, and so on. Maternity wards began implementing nurseries where babies could be cared for while mothers recovered. Basically, as soon as baby was born, they were cleaned and whisked away—cue all those movie montages of proud dads gazing through a large window into a room of bassinets, pointing happily at their little bundle. My own dad remembers staring through a nursery window, looking for my nametag, trying to figure out which red-faced little squish was me. (He should have known. I was the one who was "too pretty to be a boy.")

In the late 1970s, "new" (if you want to call "the way we had always done it across human history" new, that is) approaches to the moments after birth were in the air. Right around the same time, researchers in Sweden and the US published studies around maternal–infant bonding, focusing on SSC between mother and newborns after birth, though the phrase itself was first used in 1979 in a study out of McGill University. In the early '80s, through the pioneering work of a team of Colombian neonatal doctors, SSC, also known as "Kangaroo Care," came into widespread recognition as a vital element of the birth process. Working in an underfunded hospital with both too few nurses and too few incubators, the doctors were desperate for a solution to increase the survival rate of the preterm babies born there—a rate that stood at only 30 percent. Mothers, who were previously discouraged from visiting the NICU, were increasingly encouraged to hold their preterm infants directly against their chests for multiple hours a day. The results were staggering. Not only did these infants survive, they began to thrive. In 1983, the physicians, Edgar Rey Sanabria and Héctor Martínez-Gómez, published a study on their work, showing that SSC could benefit all babies. This finding became increasingly accepted (and researched) even in the most conventional medical settings.

Although SSC is now widely practiced at hospitals across the US, it is literally a rule at "Baby-Friendly Hospitals," one of the "Ten Steps of Successful Breastfeeding" that comprise the broad framework of the Baby-Friendly Hospital Initiative. What are "Baby-Friendly" hospitals? (I mean, who wants to give birth at a Baby-Unfriendly Hospital?) Back in 1991, the WHO and UNICEF jointly developed a plan to encourage breastfeeding, at the institutional level. Until then, many birth facilities had protocols that were not friendly to breastfeeding at all, like allowing formula marketing and advertising in the hospital and separating moms and babies after birth. Baby-Friendly Hospitals, on the other hand, undergo a rigorous credentialing process and commit to following the ten-step plan to encourage and improve breastfeeding outcomes. Today, there are over six hundred Baby-Friendly Hospitals (BFH) in the US and over 27 percent of births take place at a BFH. One of the primary tenets of BFHs is "rooming in," or keeping the baby with mom at all times. Whether or not you give birth at a BFH, you are very likely to encounter the practice. Just like SSC, the rooming in has spread widely to hospitals that are not officially "baby friendly": between 2007 and 2015, the percentage of US hospitals with 90 percent or more of newborns rooming in for at least twenty-three hours increased from 27 percent to 51 percent.

The physically, mentally, and emotionally demanding rigors of giving birth cannot be understated. In the exhaustion that follows, rooming in can be tough on moms who have to transition straight into childcare on little to no sleep, while trying to recover physically. The purported main benefit of rooming in is improved breastfeeding outcomes. In her excellent book, *Cribsheet,* economist and "decision science" expert Emily Oster combs through the data on rooming in and determines there isn't much hard evidence to support this benefit, beyond correlation. Oster's goal here is to destigmatize asking for help and/or sending your baby to the nursery for a couple of hours if needed. As she writes, "Your hospital stay includes more support than you are likely to get at home, and sending your baby to the nursery could let you take advantage of their expert care of you and your baby. Knowing that the data is not definitively on the side of rooming in can make this an easier choice for some moms . . . In my view, the most important thing to come out of this is, if you have the option to send your kid to the nursery for a few hours and you want to do that, you shouldn't feel shame in doing so. There is no good evidence that you're disrupting your breastfeeding relationship, if that's important to you. And if you find yourself falling asleep with your baby in the bed, ask for help."

I agree with Emily. No mom should feel shame in asking for help. At the same time, if everything is going well and you feel able to do so, I believe you should do your best to keep your baby with you at all times, whether or not you elect to breastfeed. For those first few days, your baby is just getting to know you. They are getting to know your smells and sounds. You are building a foundation of trust and responsiveness to their needs from day one.

Personally, there was no way my wife and I were sending Eli to the nursery for someone else to watch on the first day of his life unless that was medically necessary. And, if it was, I was going along. Letting my baby out of my sight was not an option. When I say it out loud, it sounds crazy, I know. I couldn't fathom the thought that I may become one of those cautionary tales about a couple who takes home the wrong baby. Okay, maybe this is extreme. (It goes to show you that even I, a pediatrician, went down one of those new-parent rabbit holes I referred to earlier.) Regardless, we did keep Eli with us to be sure we knew what was happening to him at all times. We did not want to risk the unlikely, but nonetheless possible, scenario in which a well-intentioned nurse made an error, administered a medication, or performed a procedure we did not authorize. If your baby is in another room, you cannot be certain of what is transpiring. I followed Eli everywhere and I think you should do the same with your newborn too, if possible.

DELAYED CORD CLAMPING

Until recently, most obstetricians would clamp a newborn's umbilical cord pretty much immediately—within ten to fifteen seconds after delivery—blocking the flow of blood from the placenta to the baby before cutting the cord. Yet research has increasingly shown the benefits to delaying cord clamping.

Many OB/GYNs are not totally on board just yet. They should get on board, though—for full-term babies, delayed cord clamping has been shown to significantly increase blood volume: at one minute after birth, approximately 80 mL of blood has transferred from the placenta, and at three minutes, that amount has increased to 100 mL. This transfer of blood from the placenta increases a newborn's iron stores, which has been shown to reduce the risk of iron deficiency during the first year of baby's life. This is a really meaningful benefit, as iron deficiencies in infants have been linked to longer-term detrimental cognitive, motor, and behavioral outcomes. Delayed cord clamping also helps facilitate the transfer of immunoglobulins and stem cells, both of which play a vital role in tissue and organ repair. For preterm babies, the benefits are even greater, including improved circulation, greater red blood cell volume, less need for blood transfusions, and lower risk of necrotizing enterocolitis (a dangerous inflammation of the large intestine) and intraventricular hemorrhage (bleeding in spaces in the brain that contain cerebrospinal fluid, which can cause brain damage).

With delayed cord clamping, there *is* a very slight increased risk of jaundice (the more blood, the more red blood cells, the more blood cells, the more of their byproduct, bilirubin)—although jaundice is very highly monitored and easily treatable. Even the American College of Obstetricians and Gynecologists (ACOG) has come out in full support of delayed cord clamping. At this point, the question isn't really "to clamp or not to clamp?" but "how long to wait?"

The answer to that question is a little less clear. While the medical community seems to be catching up to natural-minded parents when it comes to delayed cord clamping, there still isn't consensus when it comes to the length of the delay. Many natural-minded parents advocate for delaying clamping for periods beyond a minute or longer, while most OBs who practice delayed clamping wait for thirty to sixty seconds. With Eli, we delayed for about one minute.

When it comes to the professionals, there is very little consensus. Thanks, guys! The ACOG recommends delaying thirty to sixty seconds, and the American Academy of Pediatrics (AAP) agrees. Meanwhile, the WHO suggests no less than a minute. The American College of Nurse-Midwives advises that clamping be delayed for two to five minutes after birth. And so on. Like I said, thanks, guys. Based on the available evidence, my opinion is that delaying clamping for at least a minute has the highest beneficial outcome; beyond that, the benefits are less evident. So, yes, delayed cord clamping is something I advocate. Regardless of where you fall on the crunchy-to-conventional spectrum, I don't think you need to push strongly to do it for *longer* than two minutes, especially if you're giving birth in a hospital setting, where this likely isn't feasible.

In the end, the only drawback—if you want to call it that—to delayed cord clamping is that it means there is less blood available (or possibly none at all) for cord blood banking. Spoiler alert—as you will later find out, I'm not a huge believer in cord blood banking anyway. When comparing the clear, immediate value and benefits of delayed clamping to the nebulous, fuzzy limited promise of cord blood banking, the former far outweighs the latter.

CORD BLOOD BANKING

One of the more common questions parents-to-be ask me during prenatal interviews is whether or not I recommend private cord blood banking (the storage of a child's umbilical blood in a private facility, for an ongoing fee). My short answer is no, I don't recommend it (and neither does the AAP).

But let's back up a second—what is cord blood? At birth, your newborn's placenta and umbilical cord contain blood that is rich with potentially lifesaving blood-forming stem cells. These cells are so special because they can produce all the types of cells found in blood, including immune system cells. Because of that, cord blood transplants can be used to treat diseases like leukemia, sickle-cell anemia, and lymphoma, among certain other blood, immune, and metabolic diseases.

At first blush, cord blood banking sounds like a good idea—a kind of insurance policy against potential serious illness. In practice, though, private cord blood banking is not super useful. First, when it comes to most diseases that a cord blood transplant could treat, doctors would not use a patient's own blood, due to the risk it may turn cancerous or carry the same mutations. Second, most treatments private cord blood banks tout are theoretical only. Cord blood cannot cure Alzheimer's or Parkinson's or the myriad other diseases that private banks list as potential targets for treatment; there is minimal evidence to support the promise of these therapies just yet.

So, are there any benefits right now? Except in very rare cases, not really. If you already have an older child with a disease that cord blood can treat, then it may be worth private banking the cord blood of your newborn second child, on the chance he or she is a donor match for his or her sibling. That said, the likelihood of finding a bone marrow or cord blood match from a public bank is already 29 to 79 percent (depending on ethnicity). Public banks, you say? Yes—and that brings me to my third point: *public* cord banking exists. It is free, and I encourage you to donate your baby's cord blood to one, if you feel comfortable doing so. If you choose not to donate, your child's cord will be disposed of as medical waste. Your donation not only helps further the research on future uses of cord blood, it could save lives—the vast majority of cord blood transplants are done with donations from public banks.

The bottom line is that private cord blood banking can be expensive and, at this time, most of it will sit around and go unused. To be fair, we have no idea what the future will hold, so there may be more use to cord blood at some point down the line. For that reason, if you have the means and want to do it, there is no downside, other than the cost for possibly no benefit. Private cord blood banking is a business that, like many others, preys on the fear and anxiety of new parents for profit. The peace of mind it may offer is predicated on a premise that has yet to be proven.

PLACENTA ENCAPSULATION

Sometime in the mid-2010s, placentophagy (the practice of eating one's own placenta) transitioned from the purely crunchy into the semi-woo-woo-but-mainstream world. After the birth of her second child, Kim Kardashian posted her bottle of encapsulated placenta on her socials. While it doesn't get more mainstream than a Kardashian, other famous women, such as Padma Lakshmi and Chrissy Teigen, also touted the benefits of freeze-drying your placenta, grinding it up, and encapsulating it, as a way to beat postpartum depression, increase milk supply, and generally smooth the often-bumpy road to recovery that can follow birth.

Nowadays, pretty much every doula and midwife offer the service, and labor and delivery staff are unlikely to raise an eyebrow if they see this on a birth plan. This begs the question: Should you do it?

In my opinion, no. Let me be clear: I'm not here to disparage the reproductive choices women make for themselves. Some of the moms I encounter in my practice report that they have experienced benefits from taking placenta pills. That said, when it comes to evidence-based support for the practice, it's just not there. It's not there in the studies, and it's not there in our history—something I value deeply as a natural-minded doctor who feels strongly that traditional care practices, and midwifery in particular, have much to offer.

You'll hear advocates for placentophagy claim that it was practiced as part of Traditional Chinese Medicine (TCM). This simply isn't true. Yes, small amounts of dried placenta powder are mentioned as one of many ingredients in formulations to treat certain ailments, such as impotence, kidney problems, and infertility. To my knowledge, nowhere in the *Compendium of Materia Medica,* a TCM medical text from the sixteenth century, is there a description of using the placenta for postpartum issues—and certainly never one's *own* placenta. As a practice, placentophagy does not appear in historical or anthropological records from cultures across the East and the West. Centuries of midwife and birth care from diverse cultures reflect this as well. The first modern reference to human placentophagy in medical literature comes in a 1973 letter-to-the-editor in the journal *Obstetrics and Gynecology*, from an MD who, having previously authored a study on animal placentophagy, mentions reading about it in an "underground press" (which turned out to be *Rolling Stone,* reporting on commune life . . . just goes to show what a doctor at Manhattan's Beth Israel Medical Center in 1973 considered bohemian reading material). Finally, the argument that it's "natural" because "most mammals do it" is somewhat preposterous to me. Some mammals also eat their newborns. Some eat poop. Most have pretty different reproductive cycles than humans. Moreover, they eat their placentas raw, immediately after giving birth (now *that* would be a novel line item on a birth plan) . . . not cooked, and definitely not dehydrated and ground up into little pills to be consumed for days, weeks, or months afterward.

Maybe it's time for a study on human moms eating their placenta raw right after giving birth. Are you raising your hand to volunteer for that study? That said, the research is not definitive—it's lacking, and that's part of the issue. I don't think it's a coincidence that interest in placentophagy has risen over the last fifty years, specifically in the West; it's the same time period in which birth has become increasingly medicalized and medical care itself more and more corporatized. When considered in this context, the motivation behind taking placenta pills makes a lot of sense: more women than ever are interested in natural options in health care and are more aware of and concerned about preventing and treating postpartum depression. Frankly, I don't think they get enough support on this front in conventional medical settings. We need to do a better job supporting moms in the postpartum period . . . period.

NICU

If you do have a more complex birth, or baby does experience complications such as very low birth weight, respiratory distress, birth injury, infection, or the need for extra monitoring or special treatment, what can you expect? Most likely, your baby will be taken to the hospital's neonatal intensive care unit (NICU). Not all hospitals have a NICU, so, prior to your due date, it is worth asking whether the hospital at which you are planning to deliver does. If you are at a hospital without a NICU and your baby does need that extra level of care, they will be transported by the hospital to the nearest NICU. The NICU has specialized care with much closer monitoring and potentially necessary interventions at the ready. The NICU also has a much higher ratio of staff to babies than the postpartum unit or newborn nursery. For example, instead of one nurse for every fifteen babies, a NICU might have one nurse for every one to three babies.

Some of the incredible specialists you might encounter in the NICU include neonatologists (pediatricians with extra training in caring for sick and premature babies), who may supervise your baby's overall care plan; neonatal fellows (pediatricians training to be neonatologists), who may treat your baby; neonatal nurse practitioners (nurses with specialized training in caring for sick and premature babies); respiratory therapists; physical therapists; and social workers (whose job it is to provide resources, health-care information, support, and emotional and psychological counseling to families).

Hospital Procedures

In the hours and days after your baby is born, while you're still in the hospital, you'll want to sleep, or at least rest—but you won't be able to. Every five minutes (okay, I'm being dramatic, but it *feels* that way), someone will be entering your room—a nurse, the pediatrician, your OB, a lactation consultant, an audiologist, techs, and so on. There will be a lot of poking and prodding. After Eli was born, this drove my wife, Sarah, crazy. She just wanted to go home, and barring that, she just wanted to be left alone. Knowing what to expect helped mitigate her annoyance every time the door opened and another nurse walked through.

Assuming everything is going according to standard operating procedure, here's what you can expect during that day or two you'll be in the hospital after giving birth: within a few hours of birth, the baby will be offered a vitamin K shot, antibiotic eye ointment, the hepatitis B vaccine, the respiratory syncytial virus (RSV) vaccine, a hearing screen, a heart screen, and a newborn genetics screen. If you have a boy, you will have to decide whether or not to circumcise him. Feeling lost? I got you. Ultimately, every family is different; every situation is different; and it doesn't always make sense to advocate for or against something across the board.

Everyone is unique, each situation is different, and each birth plan is your own. In large part, I wrote this book to empower expectant parents and to emphasize that there is not a one-size-fits-all approach. Rather than dictate what you should and shouldn't do, I want to equip you with information so you can make intelligent decisions that are best for you and your family. I cannot tell you what to do—in large part because I am legally prohibited from giving medical advice to someone who is not my patient—but, more important, because medical advice is useless without the most important piece of the puzzle: YOU and YOUR BELIEFS.

Furnished with this information, you must think these topics through, weigh the pros and cons, and discuss important medical decisions with your partner and your care team. As you can see, many of these questions just create more questions—even for me. There is no crystal ball and we don't have data to support every specific question you may have. You should, however, look through the existing data to get a bird's-eye view on the major topics you will encounter as a new parent.

By now you have probably realized I am a natural-minded practitioner and parent. Not woo-woo or too far out there, I grew up without much knowledge of anything holistic. Heck, while I haven't touched the stuff in probably twenty years, I used to eat fast food all the time while away at hockey tournaments.

In prenatal interviews, when I meet with parents that are opposed to most medical interventions, I often mention how much higher the mortality rates used to be for babies and women in childbirth to remind my very natural-minded families that medicine is not "all bad," even if the internet says so. This is especially true in the areas of birth and the newborn period. Let's jump back to the not-so-distant past. In the early 1900s, for every thousand live births, six to nine women in the United States died of pregnancy-related complications, and approximately a hundred infants died before reaching a year old. But by 1997, those rates had declined by greater than 90 percent for infant mortality and almost 99 percent for maternal mortality.

Vitamin K is a great example of a medical leap forward. All babies are born with "low" levels of vitamin K, putting them at risk for vitamin K deficiency bleeding, which, though rare, can be life threatening. When discussing whether or not vitamin K should be part of their birth plan, parents will often ask: "Why would a baby be born deficient in something? If a baby was meant to have more vitamin K, nature would have done that." In the strictest of senses, I agree. A low level of vitamin K at birth is "natural." But babies are also born with immune systems that are not yet fully developed—and we take care to protect them, despite the fact that being born with an immature immune system is also "natural." Pneumonia is also "natural," but if you caught pneumonia before the advent of penicillin, you had a 30 to 40 percent likelihood of dying from it. For most people today, though, you can pop a few pills and be back to your oat-milk latte within days. We have undeniably come a long way in medicine in the "saving your life department."

At the same time, we cannot definitively know the long-term risks of all interventions; we must humbly admit that we are still learning. For many issues, there is no simple one-size-fits-all solution. Certain decisions are unavoidably complex, and it is important to think them through. Extremes are rarely the answer.

NEWBORN SCREENINGS

The newborn screening identifies rare conditions like sickle cell, cystic fibrosis, and other genetic, endocrine, and metabolic disorders, as well as hearing loss and congenital heart defects, that can be life threatening or cause severe consequences for long-term health. Catching these conditions early is critical—for example, with the metabolic disorder galactosemia, the body is unable to break down and process the milk sugar galactose. As galactose builds up in the body, it is converted to galactitol, a toxic alcohol derivative. Galactosemia can cause sepsis, liver failure, cognitive and developmental delays, and infertility, among a host of other devastating side effects. Remember how I just said galactose is a milk sugar? Well, it's not limited to dairy foods—it's present in breast milk too. The treatment for galactosemia is pretty obvious: avoid consuming anything that contains galactose. For a newborn whose primary source of food is breast milk, it is critical to know ASAP that this is an issue.

Genetic, Endocrine, and Metabolic Disorders Screen

Most of the conditions newborn screening is designed to catch are tested for using a few drops of blood. About twenty-four hours after your baby is born, a health-care provider will prick their heel one time and send the sample to a lab. Most parents are understandably concerned about pain from the poke. The nurse would generally be using a lancet like you would think of for diabetes. It honestly doesn't really hurt. You basically don't feel it. Trust me, I have tried it on myself. Occasionally, babies do cry. Mostly this is due to the pressure from the nurse's grip on the foot and not the prick itself.

For such a quick, simple process, the newborn screening heel prick is a pretty incredible tool for saving lives and improving health outcomes. About 12,500 newborns each year are diagnosed with one of the conditions detected through newborn screening. This means that almost 1 in every 300 newborns screened is eventually diagnosed. It's really important to note here that newborn screening itself is not diagnostic. It doesn't confirm whether or not a newborn has a disease; it *does*, however, identify that they are at risk for it. If the screen comes back positive, you'll be referred to a specialist for diagnostic tests and counseling. While different states test for different conditions, the Department of Health and Human Services does recommend universal testing for thirty-five conditions. This list is called the Recommended Uniform Screening Panel.

While all states mandate newborn screening as a matter of law to protect babies and catch treatable conditions (and most states report participation of 99.9 percent or higher), some do allow parents to opt out for religious or other reasons. I most definitely do *not* suggest opting out of screening. I mention it only because you may be wondering whether you need a newborn screening when you previously underwent genetic screening. The answer is a resounding yes. First, what most parents think of as genetic screening is technically *carrier* screening. That means you and/or your partner took a test to find out if you are carriers of certain genes, and therefore at risk of passing those genes to your child. People who do carrier testing usually do so because they belong to an ethnic group with high rates of certain diseases, or because they know they have a family history of certain diseases and disorders. The classic example of people who benefit from carrier screening is Ashkenazi Jews—there are more than nineteen recessive conditions that are more common in these individuals than in non-Ashkenazi folks. Carrier screening tests the risk of *the parent or parents* for passing along a disease. It helps would-be parents early in their pregnancy to make decisions for the best potential quality of life for their future child.

In contrast, newborn screening tests *the infant itself.* While there is some overlap between the conditions the tests screen for, the newborn screen is the one that identifies the risk for serious conditions in a baby who has just been born. Additionally, whereas carrier screening looks only for genetic issues, newborn screening looks for genetic, hormonal, and metabolic issues (like galactosemia). A prenatal genetic screening might not reveal risk for diseases or disorders under either of these categories.

Technically, even babies born at home are required by law to have newborn screening. Since the newborn screen is essentially a simple blood test done by heel prick and sent to a lab, many midwives and birth centers are trained to perform it. Before you give birth, ask your provider whether he or she is able to do this. If not, you may schedule a newborn screening at a clinic or hospital, regardless of whether or not you gave birth there.

Hearing Screen

Newborns are also tested for congenital hearing loss, which is more common than you might think—almost 2 in 1,000 babies are born deaf or hard of hearing. In addition, 90 percent of babies with hearing loss are born to two hearing parents, which can render the condition all the more unexpected. Catching hearing loss early is critical, as hearing is directly linked to language, speech acquisition, and development, especially in the first two years of life. The good news is that there are many early interventions that now exist to improve the outcomes of children with hearing loss (babies as young as six days old have been fitted with hearing aids), as well as effective ongoing supports.

CIRCUMCISION

Circumcision—the removal of the foreskin from a baby boy's penis—is incredibly common in the United States. As of 2010, about 58 percent of newborn boys, and about 80 percent of males between ages fourteen and fifty-nine were circumcised. But the decision to circumcise your child remains an intensely personal choice, especially given that in most circumstances it's not medically necessary—not to mention that it has become one of the most controversial topics in pediatrics. As a pediatrician, my goal is to help you understand both the benefits and risks of circumcision, and how to then weigh them in the context of your own familial, religious, and cultural beliefs and practices—so you can make the decision that's right for you, without guilt, fear, or worry. Tall order, I know, particularly given that, in the current landscape, everyone seems to feel the need to tell you what is best. I'll cut right to it (pun intended): this decision is up to you. Some parents are for this, and others are very against it. I'll take the pressure off: there is no wrong decision. How can that be? Medically, the benefits are minor and the risks are low. Although it is on the decline culturally—between the 1980s and 2010s, circumcisions dropped 10 percent nationally—circumcision remains common in the US. This means that no matter what you elect to do, your son is likely to see other boys who look like him.

There are a few undeniable minor benefits to circumcision. While those benefits may be statistically significant—in other words, good studies have shown that the observed data (the benefits) are unlikely to be the result of chance but, instead, are attributable to a specific cause (circumcision)—in real life, the numbers they represent are quite small. The best example of this is the number-one benefit of circumcision: lower rates of urinary tract infections. In uncircumcised boys under age two, the risk of UTIs is about 1 percent, while the risk decreases to about 0.1 percent in circumcised boys. This is a real and meaningful difference statistically: uncircumcised boys under two are ten times more likely to get a UTI than a circumcised boy. These statistics may also be viewed in a different way: to prevent just one case of UTI, you'd have to circumcise over a hundred boys. In the real world, while unfun, UTIs are seldom a big deal and so the results, although technically significant, are not strong enough evidence in my mind to recommend circumcision to all.

Admittedly, in my personal clinical experience, I have had more medical consultations about "penis stuff" with families of uncircumcised babies than with those of circumcised ones. It's never anything serious—mostly minor infections or irritation under the foreskin. Yet such encounters are few and far between.

Circumcision is one of the most widely performed procedures in the world: about one in three men is circumcised worldwide. Given this frequency, we can guess that those who perform circumcision have a lot of experience doing so; perhaps this accounts, at least in part, for its low risk of complications: in the first five years after the surgery, the rate of complications for hospital-performed circumcision is about 1.5 percent.

Among these complications, the most common include bleeding and infection. Fortunately, most bleeding in these cases is mild and can be resolved with the application of pressure and a gauze pad, or a special gel-based wrap that promotes blood clotting. Infection is a possibility with any surgery, of course. Given that most circumcisions are done in a semi-sterile setting, this outcome is rare.

Adhesions, scar tissue that forms when the skin on the shaft of the penis adheres to the glans of the penis, are also one of the more prevalent complications. Adhesions will often resolve over time, but if they do not, they can be treated with steroid cream. Inadequate foreskin removal is another risk. When either too little or too much is snipped, the child may require revision surgery.

Finally, I have to address the elephant in the room. Many people who oppose circumcision do so (at least partly) on the grounds that it reduces sensitivity and later sexual pleasure. Very limited research has been done on this topic, and with mixed results. It's tough to run any good studies on this since most rely on self-assessment, and because it's kind of impossible to report on a comparison you're not anatomically able to make (i.e., a circumcised man has no way of knowing how it feels to be uncircumcised and vice versa). Furthermore, sexual experience is undeniably highly subjective. Often, pleasure is related less to anatomy and more to psychology. The results of a small study out of Queens University in Ontario (where I did my master's in epidemiology) that involved subjecting volunteers to sensory testing (yes, zapping their bits with heat. Who volunteered for this? I hope they were paid well) challenged the idea that the foreskin is the most sensitive part of the penis. The researchers recommended further study of the relationship between the perception of pleasure and the perception of sensation.

If you do choose to circumcise, the first step is to make sure everything is okay anatomically and in proper working order. Once that's confirmed, you must decide where to have the circumcision performed. Most circumcisions are performed in the hospital by an OB within a day or two of birth, but traditionally, for Jewish families, circumcision is done on the eighth day of the infant's life, in an at-home ceremony called a bris. At a bris, a mohel (a person specially trained in the rite of circumcision) will perform the operation. Sometimes circumcision is done outside the hospital, but in a medical setting, like a pediatrician's or urologist's office.

Regardless of where it's done or by whom, pain relief should absolutely be used. The myth that newborns cannot feel pain is just that—a myth. You do have the option of an injection nerve block or giving some alcohol, like wine. Following a circumcision, not much is required of you. Immediately after, keep the area clean and dry with the diaper off. For a few days thereafter, cover the area with cream or lotion and gauze, with the diaper on. Have it checked by your doctor, but otherwise, it should heal up within a week or two.

Weighing both the benefits and the risks of circumcision, the AAP has come out in support of circumcision as beneficial to male babies, stopping short of actually recommending it as a routine procedure. Acknowledging that it is a non-necessary, elective medical procedure, the AAP's official stance is that parents should have access to it and that insurance should cover it, but that ultimately parents need to make the decision for themselves. And now we've come full circle—back to the controversy. At its heart, this controversy is about the ethics of circumcision, about consent. Circumcision does permanently alter the body, and of course, newborns cannot consent to it. A patient's informed consent must be a foundational principle of any medical doctor's practice. Of course, this is far trickier for a pediatrician. Afterall, minor children cannot legally give consent and parents or guardians are tasked with the responsibility of making medical decisions for them. Both pediatricians and parents have an ethical duty to act in the *best interest* of the child. When it comes to circumcision, medically and in terms of health outcomes, both choices are legitimate.

Reasonable people can disagree. Yet, in determining what constitutes *the best interest* of a child overall, part of that consideration is going to be cultural. What I would discourage parents from doing is making the choice to circumcise "just because." I encourage you to speak with your pediatrician or OB and to weigh the benefits and risks in the context of your own family—how important are the traditions of your religion to you? Will choosing to circumcise or not affect your child's ability to participate in your religious community? How much does it matter to you that your child look like his father, or like most other American boys (for now)? How comfortable and committed will you be to teaching your child how to care for their body, should you choose not to circumcise? If you want to defer the decision until your child can consent, do you accept that the risks of circumcision are greater the older the age at which it is performed? As you ask yourself these questions, your answers might lead you in a direction you didn't expect, and that's okay. What matters is that your decision will be thoughtful and informed, which is *always* in the best interest of your child.

Most-Common Newborn Concerns

WEIGHT LOSS

During the first few days of your baby's life, your doctors, nurses, and midwives will be actively monitoring your child for weight loss and jaundice—two of the most common newborn issues, which often go hand in hand. When it comes to weight, nurses will weigh baby about every twelve hours. Why? In the beginning, many babies are not that great at feeding. They're obviously new to the world. They're not, you know, magically perfect at sucking straight out of the gate. (We had the opposite problem. Eli was a voracious eater who went straight for the boob and didn't want to let go. Thus, it came as no surprise when he went on to savor food more than any child I have ever seen. With his discerning and sophisticated palate, we call him a baby gourmand . . . but these are stories befitting of another book.) At first, mom doesn't produce a lot of milk. It can take up to seventy-two hours for milk to come in; prior to that your baby may just be getting a few drops of colostrum—the nutrient-dense earliest breast milk, high in antibodies and antioxidants to build a newborn baby's immune system—at every feeding. This may prove confounding to many parents. On top of this reduced calorie consumption (compared to life in the womb), breastfeeding is hard work. Think of it as newborn aerobics.

This trifecta leads to initial weight loss in that first week of life. We expect to see babies lose anywhere from 5 percent up to 10 percent of their birth weight. After the first week, we expect babies to gain half an ounce to an ounce a day and they should be back up to birth weight by about two weeks. (We'll get into what to do and what may be going on if baby is not gaining weight as expected when we venture into our deep dive on breastfeeding in section 3.) Weight loss beyond the norm is a concern because it indicates baby isn't getting enough fluids (i.e., breast milk)—and is therefore at risk of dehydration. Our bodies need plenty of fluid to make blood and for our cells and organs to function properly. Consequently, dehydration in newborns is a serious concern. If your baby does experience disconcerting weight loss, your doctor will likely recommend supplementation (though not usually before forty-eight hours). I know a lot of parents are anxious that supplementation will interfere with breastfeeding, but there is no hard evidence to support this. I am a strong proponent of breastfeeding wherever possible, but when a baby's health is at risk, sometimes the right thing to do is supplement with formula or donor breast milk in the short term. As breastfeeding improves, you can ditch the supplementation, should you choose to do so. Health is a priority, though, regardless of your birth plan. Sometimes plans change; parenting requires constant flexibility and pivots. Ensuring your baby gets enough to eat and preventing dehydration are of the utmost importance. In order to better understand whether or not your child's weight loss is within range (and to help inform your decision about supplementing), you can use a tool, developed by doctor-researchers at Penn State and the University of California, to determine how your newborn's weight in the first days of life compares to a large sample of newborns (see the Recommended Resources on page 249 for more information).

JAUNDICE

Monitoring a newborn's weight can also help identify babies at greater risk of developing jaundice (which usually appears on day two or three). Jaundice is a condition in which excess levels of bilirubin build up in the blood, causing yellowing of the skin and eyes. As red blood cells break down, they produce bilirubin. Normally, the liver processes the bilirubin and passes it, in bile, into the gut. Our digestive system then eliminates it as part of our waste matter. That's right, it gets pooped and peed out. Newborn babies who aren't doing much eating are also not doing much pooping or peeing. In this situation, the bilirubin hangs out in the gut too long and gets reabsorbed into the bloodstream. Newborns are also more susceptible to jaundice because their livers are not fully mature. Not only are their livers not as efficient at processing bilirubin, but on top of this, they are breaking down a higher amount of red blood cells, creating a greater strain on their already immature livers.

Jaundice is relatively common—up to 60 percent of newborns experience some degree of jaundice. Most won't require treatment; as they feed more and, accordingly, pee and poop more, the jaundice will fade on its own (in about a week for formula-fed babies and two to three weeks for breastfed babies). A typical experience in the hospital goes like this: Feeding did not go perfectly on day one. Little Emma is still working on her suck and has peed just once. The doctor encourages mom to have a lactation consult. Twenty-four hours after birth, the doctor informs mom that the jaundice levels in the baby are at a moderate level of concern. Over the next day, the feeding improves and the doctor checks your baby's blood two times. The bilirubin levels are no longer in the concerning range and you are sent home with a follow-up "jaundice check" with your pediatrician in two days.

The danger occurs when bilirubin levels become *too* high—excess bilirubin can lead to a kind of brain damage called kernicterus, which can cause cerebral palsy, hearing loss, vision loss, and intellectual disabilities. The good news is that kernicterus is extremely rare these days, as newborns' bilirubin levels are very carefully monitored if they get higher than we would like (usually through heel prick blood testing) and because treatment is readily available. Phototherapy—where your baby will lie in a bassinet, wearing only a diaper and eye protectors, under special lights that help break down bilirubin—is easy and noninvasive.

If you leave the hospital in fewer than seventy-two hours after your baby's birth (three days), you'll need to have baby checked again within the next few days.

Leaving the Hospital

CAR SEATS

Time moves very strangely in a hospital, especially after giving birth. It can shift unexpectedly from crystal clear to blurry and back again. It makes perfect sense, really. The incessant sleep interruptions, lack of natural light, and residual effects of any pain management leave you discombobulated and exhausted. Nevertheless, whether you've been there for one day or one week, the time has come: you are being released, with a terrifyingly fragile newborn in your arms. So why is this section called "Car Seats" and not just "Leaving the Hospital"? Because you can't leave the hospital without a car seat.

Here's the thing: all infant car seats in the United States have to meet certain federally regulated safety standards. As long as you are buying a new seat (I suggest avoiding used seats, since it is more difficult to know if they have been involved in an accident previously or if they meet current safety standards), from a reputable retailer, and the seat is clearly labeled, it's inherently safe. If, before your bundle of joy arrives, you're feeling stressed with baby prep, spend less time researching seven million car seats. Ultimately, they all have relatively similar safety standards. Instead, make sure the seat you buy will fit in your car *and that it's installed correctly.* There you have it. You're welcome.

Correctly installing a car seat is much more difficult than most new parents realize. It's not that putting in car seats is intellectually or physically hard, but getting the angle and incline right, while making sure it's also properly secured, is deceptively tricky, given the variety of car seats and the variety of cars out there. People who install car seats professionally are required to take a two-week-long course on how to do it, because there are so many different variables.

Even though I'm a pediatrician (or because I am one), Sarah and I still went to our local car seat installation business and had our car seat inspected. They showed us how to adjust it, made the adjustments, reviewed proper use of the restraints and harness, and sent us on our merry way with invaluable peace of mind and much more confidence in what we were doing. Besides the safety of your child, the lessened worry and anxiety itself is priceless.

Finally, consider purchasing a "travel system." This is a car seat/stroller combo affair. The car seat clips in and out of a base in the car, and then in and out of a compatible stroller frame. They are so, so useful because they mean you can move a sleeping baby in and out of the car without waking them. They are also great if you use multiple cars or have family members or caregivers who will be driving with baby. Instead of purchasing two or more car seats, you can purchase extra bases and install those in grandma's or the nanny's car, which is much more cost-effective. Travel systems themselves can be a little more expensive than separate car seats and strollers, but they have the added value of their flexibility, which is worth the additional cost and those extra hours of sleep your baby will get. Trust me, you're going to appreciate every second of extra sleep your baby gets, so an extra fifty or hundred bucks may be worth it. There are many options that are budget friendly. You don't have to buy the Rolls-Royce of travel systems. This is also a good gift to put on your registry—you could even list it as an item that multiple people can purchase as a group. Alternatively, if a grandparent or family member would like to make a more generous purchase, this may be the perfect gift. Of all the newborn purchases, this is probably the one you will use most. While spending top dollar on useless baby products is not justified, splurging on the travel system is.

IT'S NORMAL

Before we embark on that next potentially panic-inducing step—bringing baby home—I will leave you with quite possibly the most valuable wisdom I've learned from my years in pediatric practice: out of every hundred worried calls and texts I get from new parents, there is possibly *one* that requires further action. That's right, *one*. My job is basically to tell parents "it's normal" and "it's okay." That's what I'm paid the theoretical big bucks to do (pediatricians don't actually make the big bucks in medicine . . . I probably should have gone into orthopedic surgery, or worked for pharma or an insurance company). Some days, I feel I should just hire a guy to stand outside my office holding a sign that reads, "It's normal," and save everyone the copay. The truth is that our new parent brains skew the odds. When it comes to our babies, we are programmed to focus on the "what ifs." And that *is* important, because sometimes we absolutely do need to worry. But 99.9 percent of the time, you don't need to be so concerned.

Remember, if you find yourself worrying late at night about whether an issue is normal, it most likely is. While it doesn't hurt to double-check with your doctor, it's essential to keep worries in perspective. Most of the time, you can take solace in the reminder "it's normal." Parents have an innate sense of what's right for their child, built from countless interactions and observations. Trusting this intuition, combined with the knowledge gained from experience, can empower you to recognize that you frequently possess deeper insights than you give yourself credit for.

I'll say it again: *you got this.*

SECTION II

Coming Home

Congratulations! You've navigated the hospital stay, and it's time to bring your precious newborn home. This transition from a controlled, clinical setting to your own home can feel both exhilarating and nerve-wracking. While the hospital staff provided a safety net of sorts, you're now tasked with complete responsibility for your infant's care. In this section, we'll explore the essential holistic approaches to ease your transition and facilitate a nurturing home environment. From understanding what stuff you may need in the nursery to postpartum blues, I will equip you with the integrative strategies and information needed to alleviate the stressors intrinsic to this transitional phase. Welcome home.

Visitors

Even though newborn babies do little more than sleep, eat, and poop, many people can't get enough of them—especially when they're not the parent of the baby. I don't know what it is about newborns that compels the onslaught of would-be visitors. Maybe it's some need to celebrate a weird primal relief that *Hurray! The survival of our species is secured anew!* or just the almost hypnotic fact of their tininess and the inability to believe we were ever that small. Whatever it may be, the arrival of a newborn means the clamoring of folks who want to hold, coo over, and (oh no) kiss the baby. These might be grandparents, in-laws, family, coworkers, neighbors, a high school Facebook friend you forgot about after your last login in 2020, or a random relative whose position in the schema of cousins you can't quite figure out. It's overwhelming when everyone you know starts coming out of the woodwork to meet your newborn. You can and should draw boundaries.

Let's start with the simplest fact, which is that newborns' immune systems are not fully developed. During the first three months of life (which you'll hear referred to as "the fourth trimester," for good reason), newborns are more prone to infection. Their blood-brain barrier is not fully developed either, rendering them more susceptible to serious, severe, and life-threatening infection. *All* visitors must take basic precautions: wash their hands on arrival, refrain from kissing the baby, and limit the duration of the visit. If they are sick or have the slightest sniffle, they should be asked to stay home. It also doesn't hurt to ask yourself if you trust this person to be honest with you/with themselves. I cannot tell you how many times a terrified parent has come into my office, kicking themselves for not trusting their gut when a friend or relative said, "It's just allergies!" only for the guest to call later in the day, announcing he or she came down with a fever or worsening symptoms.

Hear this loud and clear (YES, I'M YELLING): "allergies" are not welcome in your home in the first few weeks. Maybe they *are* seasonal allergies, but maybe those "allergies" will turn out to be a respiratory virus—you never know. When you have a newborn baby, you can't play it too safe. It's not worth the week of fear and the potential hospital visit, as well as feeling like you screwed up and exposed your newborn to a deadly disease. The first few weeks are tough enough. Don't let someone in your home who is not 100 percent healthy. DON'T DO IT.

Consider what's most important to you in this new phase of life and what will continue to matter after this phase (the newborn period) passes. If you are really close with your family, then by all means invite your parents and siblings to come by if that is meaningful to you. No matter how badly that second cousin, twice removed, wants to meet baby, consider whether now is really the time to invite him or her, or whether waiting a few months may be the safer and better idea. Don't be afraid to be selfish and keep your stress levels low. I don't mean post a set of rules and requirements to social media detailing the terms of crossing your threshold (we've all seen those cringe inducing Reddit "Am I the A**hole" posts). I do mean ban looky-loos for the time being. Anyone who doesn't need to be around shouldn't be around. Ask the people who do come over to help you. Remember, your job for now is to prioritize your well-being so that you can best take care of your baby during a destabilizing time that will demand more of you than little else has.

If you need some backup, blame your doctor. Heck, blame me. I always tell my patients to let me be the bad guy. If the in-laws are going to make your life miserable, you aren't going to have the energy to deal with it. Let your family know that your amazing pediatrician recommended limiting visitors for two months. I'm perfectly okay taking the blame on this one.

The Business of Baby Stuff

Chances are, if you're getting ready to have a baby, you might have put together a registry or plan on putting one together. At the very least, you've probably scrolled some social media accounts that showcase "Woodland Theme" nurseries, camp-style pennants lettered with baby's name, minimalist cribs, Moses baskets, gallery walls of baby animal portraits, outer space mobiles . . . I could go on. These kinds of accounts and the influencers who run them do a really amazing job of prettifying having a baby. They rarely show a mom in a stained nursing bra, hospital-issued giant plastic water bottle on the side table, pumping or breastfeeding, or a dad in grungy sweats on his seventh lap around the living room (carefully navigating the swing, the play gym, the pump, old takeout on the coffee table), baby in arms, desperately trying to tame the worst of witching hour. There is an unspoken promise in these images of new parenthood served up in our timelines—that if you buy this stuff, that if you organize the nursery in this way (which already presumes you need a nursery), having a newborn will be as soft-focused, gentle, and beautiful—as easy—as it looks for these parents. And that's not to mention the straightforward targeted ads, many of which are just as, if not more, savvy and compelling than the "content" they punctuate, selling vibrating cradles, high-tech cameras, heart rate and oxygen monitors, luxury diapers, you name it. Any gadget, device, or thing that they promise will not only make life easier but, more important, offer *control.* They will banish fear and keep baby safe.

Look, I get it. Having a baby is crazy exciting and planning for baby's arrival by collecting all of this new stuff can be a lot of fun, not to mention make it feel more "real." However, this can quickly spiral into unhealthy perfectionism and ridiculous expectations we set for ourselves, driven by the messaging and advertisements around new parenthood. There are so many ostensible boxes to check—car seats, strollers, cribs, clothes, decorations, the right books, the right toys—and checking them will mean you're ready, right? The nursery must be finished and it has to be perfect before you bring home that bundle of joy. There's so much unspoken pressure on parents. You're already so stressed when you're having a baby and you're already thinking about being a good parent and how to do everything. The one thing you *can* do (in the face of all you can't control or do yet) is buy stuff. There's this pervasive idea that if you have everything ready, you're on the first step of being good parents. It's like, you've got the nursery, you've got everything, and you're ready to be a parent—and a *great* one.

Buying things does not make you a good parent (or a "bad" parent, though I don't like to think in those terms). Not only is the pressure to do so unfair, especially for families of limited means, or who are more frugal, it's rooted in a lie. I don't know how else to put it. It's kind of like the "dream wedding" and the wedding industrial complex (my wife wrote a book on this topic). The whole enterprise is designed to get people to spend money. And people lose sight of what really matters. There's just an endless bombardment of baby gear advertising designed to make us feel like all of these different things are not just nice to have, but *necessary.* First of all, almost none of the stuff you're told is indispensable or life changing is actually necessary or all that helpful. Most of the time, newborn babies don't sleep in their own room anyway (the AAP recommends parents keep babies in the room with them until at least six months—more on that shortly). A new baby is unlikely to use his or her nursery *for half a year or more* after being brought home. Getting everything done before the baby comes should not be your goal.

There are people all over the world that don't have a lot of stuff who will be great parents, right? We know this. So what do you need? We talked about car seats already. At home, you need a place where baby can sleep safely. It doesn't have to be a fancy crib, or even a crib at all. It could be a bassinet (though after baby reaches twenty pounds, the AAP recommends switching to a crib). In Finland, which has the lowest rate of infant mortality in the world, all expectant mothers are provided with a cardboard box of necessities, including a mattress that fits in the box, which is then used as a crib. Yes, you heard me right: many Finnish newborns sleep in cardboard boxes, and they are thriving. You need diapers and wipes and a tube of diaper cream, just in case. Again, in terms of what's necessary, not what's nice to have, you can change your baby on a towel on your bed, on the floor, you don't *need* a changing table or a $200 peanut-shaped changing pad. Diaper bins, swaddles—nice to haves, not need to haves.

You need to feed your baby, and to be prepared in case breastfeeding doesn't go as planned, or you can't or are choosing not to breastfeed. This means a few bottles, formula, and a pump (almost all insurance will cover a pump; you can get it while you're pregnant and have it available when the baby comes home from the hospital). All that other stuff—like bottle and wipe warmers, formula dispensers/mixers, bottle sanitizers—none of those are necessary. Whether or not they even make life easier is debatable, but that's up to you. Personally, I find they often take up valuable counter space and create another set of tiny parts and pieces that need to be hand washed . . . I'm definitely not a fan of adding chores to the plate of new parents.

You need something for baby to wear—a few sets of newborn onesies will probably suffice, and a few in the next two larger sizes. (Pro tip: many babies outgrow newborn clothes pretty much immediately, so you might not need them for long. Don't overdo it on the newborn size. Most get there within a few weeks. Some are born bigger than newborn size already.) Honestly, these should just be plain, inexpensive clothes you can wash over and over. As you will quickly learn, they are totally, 100 percent going to get dirty. I know, baby clothes are cute and you almost certainly need at least one outfit for the newborn photoshoot you have been waiting for! Absolutely. I'm not here telling you what *not* to buy; I'm here to bring the focus back to what is *truly necessary*, as a hard reset on our cultural conditioning.

Those are the basic musts—a place to sleep, food to eat, a way to manage poops and pees, and clothes to wear. There are obviously other useful items like a wrap or carrier, a stroller (some parents might consider this an immediate must for at least getting out to take a walk, but again it's not strictly necessary especially at first), a bathtub for baby, pacifiers, burp cloths (or you can just throw a dish towel over your shoulder), and so on.

My point is, it doesn't take a lot of stuff to bring a newborn home. You're still a great parent without the trappings of the baby industrial complex. And as you do think about what you need, or just what you want, what would be nice to have, remember: your baby doesn't care if they are sleeping in a thousand-dollar crib from Sweden, or a cardboard box. Many parents I've known got the expensive, fancy electronic bassinet that vibrates and promises to soothe your child to sleep, but ended up using it once. The motions didn't work for their baby, or they ended up feeling the cost didn't justify the benefits and sent it back. If you can afford one and want to go for it, there's no harm to your baby (although I do wonder about the possible effects of all the Wi-Fi and Bluetooth signals so close to a newborn baby for extended periods of time in some of these chichi bassinets, but that's a discussion for another day). When it comes to your wallet, you'll have to make that call. For us, we chose a simple bassinet. No movement. No gizmos. Definitely no Wi-Fi.

Although I am not opposed to superfluous and costly baby gizmos and gadgets, there is one product I believe does more harm than good. Specifically, monitors/pulse oximeters that track baby's heart rate and oxygenation level generally cause *more* unnecessary stress for parents of healthy newborns. Unless there is some medical need to strap a pulse oximeter to a newborn's foot during sleep (in which case the baby would likely be at the hospital), these devices typically take a toll on a parent's mental health. Most babies' oxygen levels rise and fall over the course of a night. This means you're going to get a lot of beeping that isn't indicative of anything. They create a lot of false alarms, as they tend to fall off frequently or come loose. A majority of parents I know who have invested in one of these devices have done so in hopes of preventing sudden infant death syndrome (SIDS) (for more on SIDS, see page 62). After all, that is the implicit promise of the device: rest easy knowing that if your baby stops breathing, you'll be alerted. Unfortunately, as far as I know, there is no evidence that shows these devices prevent SIDS—and the AAP actively recommends against using them for this purpose, stating, "Do not use home cardiorespiratory monitors as a strategy to reduce the risk of SIDS. Use of cardiorespiratory monitors has not been documented to decrease the incidence of SIDS." The AAP has expressed concern that "use of these monitors will lead to parent complacency and decreased adherence to safe sleep guidelines." I agree with the AAP on this one. Spend your hard-earned dollars elsewhere.

Will We Ever Sleep Again?

PARENT SLEEP

This is a book about babies and toddlers, yes. But when it comes to what to know or what to expect with newborn sleep (or the lack thereof), really the first thing to understand is how intense its effects will be on YOU. It's a cruel joke that just as you embark on one of the most life-altering journeys a person can experience, you also join a club that no one wants to belong to: the fellowship of the sleep deprived. Membership perks include compromised emotional regulation, brain fog, tears, and sheer all-consuming exhaustion. Unless you've had a baby before—or done some time with shift work—you're not prepared for it. Even if you *have*, you're still not prepared for it (it's like labor pain . . . the memories go hazy, probably as a mechanism to ensure the survival of our species, otherwise, seriously, who would do it again—let alone over and over?). I remember thinking the thirty-hour shifts I worked during residency were the worst sleep deprivation I would ever experience in my life. I hated the sleepless nights more than anything. It was my least favorite part of medical training and it made me consider quitting on many occasions. I didn't feel in my right mind and I don't think that doctors or anyone should ever be expected to work that long. Without the reasonable sleep needed to function, you can't fly a plane, but you can perform surgery? Makes perfect sense. Having a child took me straight back to my medical training days.

I'm really not into the "disaster parenting" content that's almost as prevalent as the sunset-tinted toddler content cluttering up social media, and I definitely don't think scaremongering is an effective tool for promoting good health. However, the sleep deprivation is real, and damn, it's hard. The best thing you can do for yourself and your baby is accept and understand *ahead of time* that you are not going to sleep a lot after you bring your newborn home, and you're not going to sleep well—probably for a little while. Prepare your life for this fact as best as you can. Rest assured (an admittedly terrible choice of words for this section), it won't last forever. While it may seem like an eternity in that sleep deprived moment, you will sleep again in a relatively short amount of time.

There have been more studies than I can count on the links between lack of sleep and mental health, as well as emotional regulation. When we don't get enough sleep, we're much more susceptible to anxiety and depression (and, how fun is this, it's a neat little circle: anxiety and depression make it harder to sleep well). Just one night of crappy sleep can seriously affect one's mood, shorten your fuse, and make you more irritable, angry, and likely to snap. Without rest, your poor brain just can't keep everything in check, allowing the amygdala (the emotional center of the brain) to wild out. Reactivity becomes the name of the game. Lack of sleep also causes brain fog and physical exhaustion, making it harder to think clearly, make decisions, and execute daily tasks.

All of this stuff is probably going to hit hardest at around a month, when you've accumulated a pretty significant sleep debt and you're deep in what can be the monotony of very early parenthood. I see every baby I care for at around one month—it's one of the standard well-visit ages—and that means I see many, many parents at one month. Every single one I see appears . . . let's just say, less put-together than usual. Even for those with Hollywood-engineered, catwalk-ready good looks, the under-eye circles are dark, and the sweatpants are omnipresent. The fatigue is plain as day. And most parents express similar feelings: guilt that they're not meeting some standard of breezy new parenthood that they've seen online. You'll probably feel like you should be cooking or cleaning. You'll probably grow frustrated that these tasks seem so much harder to tend to than they used to. That's because they *are.* You are tired and doing those things is tiring. It's okay for your priorities and standards to be different right now than they were before baby. If your house is a mess, guess what? You have a whole new human to keep alive. You're working so hard already. I have not been to a house visit for a newborn yet where one parent doesn't apologize for the mess. Even in the Hollywood Hills mega mansions, which cost more money than I will probably ever make in my life, with maids and house managers and doulas, the main room the baby spends time in is still a mess. The rest of the house is probably cleaner than yours, or mine, after a baby. We can't all have a staff. Honestly, I wouldn't want staff after a new baby even if I could afford it. My wife would probably lose it without the quiet and calm of an empty house. I want that time for baby to bond with me. Try to be more accepting of the mess and clean only if you feel up to it.

Be compassionate with yourself and your partner. Remind yourself that this is all normal and very temporary. You are not alone. All parents go through this and it will not last forever. Keeping things in perspective is the best gift you can bestow on your sanity. Sleep deprivation changes how we perceive things, increasing our negativity bias. It makes us less emotionally resilient, so things can seem worse than they are. I'm not saying that your emotions are not real. They are! But for most of us, emotions are fleeting. Feelings are not forever. They are temporary, not a life sentence. Give yourself grace.

On the practical front, I know firsthand that there are few things moms like hearing less than "Sleep when the baby sleeps." (Why moms hear this more than dads is a whole different conversation.) I get it—those times that your hands are free, that you're not completely occupied with meeting someone else's needs, feel rare and precious. And they are! (And if you have twins, you probably won't have any free hands for a long while.) This seems to me a good reason not to waste those precious free moments on tasks that don't refill your emotional gas tank, like housecleaning, and do something that *will* restore you. If you can't, or choose not to, sleep, allow yourself to rest. Welcome whatever help you can get. When people ask you what they can do, don't demur. Tell them—*we could use some food, I need someone to come over and hold the baby, would you be willing to run a load of laundry for me and fold it?* Don't be an entitled jerk, but try to disabuse yourself of the notion that asking for help is wrong or rude. If you have the privilege to outsource anything, do it: laundry service, housecleaning, grocery delivery. If ever there was one, this is the moment for two-day delivery. When my sister had a baby, I flew across the country to come help. Fold laundry, play with the toddler, carry a basket of clothes, order some food. Whatever is needed, don't feel shy to ask. I wanted to help. Your family will too (hopefully). Especially if they have had a child before. They will get it. And make sure that, if you're in a two-parent household, both parents are taking night shifts, if possible. If you're bottle feeding at all (pumped breast milk or formula), share the load when it comes to night feedings.

Finally, know that there is going to come a moment when you feel like you just can't handle it anymore. This is normal. My mother-in-law recounts plopping face first onto the bed when my wife was just one month old and muttering, "I can't do it anymore." She did it. You can do it. Feeling hopeless or exasperated doesn't mean you're a bad parent, it means you're exhausted. We've all been there. While the knowledge of all this won't lessen your exhaustion in the moment, I hope it will lessen the blow, and, fingers crossed, prevent any guilt you might experience. Yes, having a child is magical, unexplainable, wonderful, yadda yadda yadda—but in the thick of a sleepless month, it can also feel like you're trapped, or that life will never be normal again. I know my wife and I felt that way for a few days. We were prepared, though, which made it slightly easier to remain optimistic. It's natural to experience negative feelings when you're carrying a heavy load and running on empty. Life will never be the same, but I swear to you: you *will* sleep again. Hang in there.

SIDS and Safe Sleep

As you watch your newborn baby sleep, a sense of awe and joy envelops you. Yet, often this ostensible peace is undermined by a foreboding anxiety. For most new parents, there is no greater fear than sudden infant death syndrome (SIDS), which can make getting the little sleep you do all the more challenging. The anxiety and fear literally keeps some parents awake. Although the most unimaginable and catastrophic outcome a parent can fathom isn't a palatable topic of conversation, a straightforward discussion is the best way to mitigate your understandable fear (and hopefully get you a little more sleep).

So, what is SIDS? SIDS is the unexplained death of an otherwise healthy infant under one year old, usually while sleeping. Babies between one and four months of age are at greatest risk for SIDS and 90 percent of incidences of SIDS happen before six months. While SIDS is the leading cause of death for infants one month to one year, it is vital, I think—beyond critical, really—to state here that the risk of SIDS is truly so small: in 2020, SIDS occurred in 38.4 per 100,000 infants in the United States.

We do not know what causes SIDS, but ongoing research does suggest that it may be caused in part by abnormalities in the area of the brain stem that controls breathing, arousal (ability to wake from sleep), heart rate, and temperature. And yet, despite the unknowns, we *do* have power when it comes to SIDS: we know how to decrease the risk. There *are* clear actions we can take to help minimize our children's susceptibility to SIDS. Nothing demonstrates this more starkly than the number one choice you can make for your child's safety when it comes to SIDS: **putting them to sleep on their back.**

In 1992, the AAP recommended—for the first time—putting children to sleep on their back, based on studies coming out of Australia, New Zealand, and the United Kingdom that were showing a significant link between sleeping in the prone position (on the tummy) and SIDS. This was actually a super-controversial position to take. Before 1992, the vast majority of babies in the US slept on their stomach—between 70 and 80 percent of infants. Dr. Spock himself was a strong proponent of putting babies to sleep on their tummy and most pediatricians recommended it.

The thinking was that babies sleep more soundly on their stomach and that doing so offered protection against choking. Here's the thing when we get down to the nuts and bolts of this topic: when I meet parents who are resistant to following the back-to-sleep guideline, it is almost always because one of their biggest fears, if not the biggest, is that their baby will choke on their saliva while sleeping. (If you hadn't previously considered this, please don't let yourself spiral down yet another rabbit hole. It's not common.) I get it. After all, what are we taught to do if someone vomits while passed out? Roll them onto their side. It seems only logical that this would be true for newborns too—or at the very least, a logical source of concern. The good news is that a baby's anatomy is actually well-designed to prevent spit-up or fluid from entering the windpipe or lungs when lying on their back. This is because gravity works in favor of keeping these substances in the stomach and esophagus, rather than allowing them to flow upward into the respiratory system. A healthy baby with normal anatomy choking to death in the back-to-sleep position is not a concern, based on numerous studies. In fact, the AAP safe sleep policy statement categorically spells this out: when babies sleep on their back, death rates decrease. The evidence for this is inescapable, as you'll soon see.

As a parent, the choice is always yours, but it's critical to weigh the evidence and make a decision that minimizes your child's overall risk. The risk of SIDS decreases when a baby sleeps on his or her back. In 2012 the National Institute of Child Health and Human Development (NICHD) launched "Safe to Sleep," with a focus on safe sleep environments for babies. As part of the campaign, the NICHD focused on "The ABCs of Safe Sleep."

A—Alone

B—on the Back

C—in an empty Crib

Alone means babies should sleep *by themselves,* that is, in their crib or bassinet, and not in the same bed as parents. Bed sharing exposes babies to an increased potential for overheating, suffocation in loose or soft bedding, entrapment, and overlay (when an adult accidentally rolls onto a baby in sleep). The latest research shows that babies who share a bed have almost three times the odds of experiencing SIDS compared to those who don't. With bed sharing, the risk was highest for infants of smoking mothers and infants less than twelve weeks old. If your child falls in either of these groups, that is all the more reason to consider the safe sleep recommendations when making choices about where you and your baby will sleep.

Caregivers should also *never* sleep with a baby in a recliner or on a sofa, which is hands down the most dangerous form of co-sleeping—the risk of sleep-related infant death is up to sixty-seven times higher when infants sleep with someone on a couch, cushion, cushioned chair, or other soft sitting surface, and ten times higher when sleeping with someone who is impaired from the use of sedating medications, alcohol, or drugs.

Now, this one is already a *no* for many obvious reasons both in terms of pregnancy and, you know, living a long and healthy life: DON'T SMOKE. I'm not here to guilt-trip you, but I am a doctor and I do care about you (or I wouldn't be writing this book). If you smoke at all, even "just socially," and have a newborn, please, please stop. Not only is smoking terrible for you in countless ways, all of which have been enumerated in a million public health campaigns, but smoking during pregnancy and by either parent after pregnancy are major risk factors for SIDS. Babies born to mothers who smoke throughout pregnancy have a fivefold increase in risk of SIDS compared to babies whose mothers have never smoked. Infants exposed to secondhand smoke are twice as likely to die of SIDS. Given the numerous studies that have shown a causal link between smoking and SIDS, many researchers now feel that in industrialized countries like the US, smoking is the greatest modifiable risk factor for SIDS—in other words, it's the number-one behavior individuals can change to lower the risk of SIDS. By some estimates, one-third of SIDS deaths could be prevented if everyone stopped smoking during and after pregnancy.

Following safe sleep practices—and avoiding risky behaviors—saves lives. That's all there is to it. But I do want to address something else here too—the reality that sometimes we all fail to meet the standards of best practices or choose not to follow the guidelines. Doing so can cause a lot of shame for parents, and this shame can make less-than-ideal situations worse. People who feel shame often hide what they feel bad about or avoid acknowledging it, meaning they miss opportunities to make better or different choices even if they can't make the theoretical best choice. What am I getting at here? Look, many parents I know or take care of bed-share with their babies. For even the best, most well-intentioned, and risk-averse parents, bed sharing can end up feeling like a matter of survival. One child might be happy to sleep in a bassinet right away. Another might not sleep unless a parent is holding him or her. You may start to feel like you won't otherwise ever get to sleep. Your baby won't be able to sleep. It's a bleak domino effect. Many parents tell me they are bed sharing at least some of the time. It's not just "crunchy" parents who engage in co-sleeping. A 2015 Centers for Disease Control and Prevention (CDC) survey of women who had recently given birth found that 61 percent of respondents self-reported bed sharing. A number of parents arrive there out of what they feel is necessity, even if they set out not to do so.

Unfortunately, though, many people who practice bed sharing may not acknowledge it or tell their pediatricians, out of shame. They know there are risks with bed sharing, such as an increased chance of SIDS, suffocation, or entrapment, and that they are "not supposed to do it." Yes, it's essential for doctors to inform parents of the best, safest way for baby to sleep based on the available research. But too often, that's *all* we tell them. We ignore reality and behave as though all other choices besides the "best" choice are equally bad—which is simply not true. To me, this is one of the most fundamental failures of modern medicine: it often lacks an acknowledgment of reality. Instead, it's more like "Here's the research. Here's what the double-blind study shows; this is what you should be doing. Don't do anything else ever." As a doctor, I feel the oath I took compels me not only to inform people of what they *must* do, but also to address what they are *actually doing*.

While, based on the data, I do not recommend bed sharing, I also believe that, if it does come to that, you should understand the increased risks, assess whether you are comfortable assuming those risks, and, if you still decide to proceed, understand the ways to minimize them as best you can. Like every choice you make for your child, you have to weigh the pros and cons in the context of your specific situation. When it comes to SIDS, if you are bed sharing, it is best not to smoke, to be on any sedative medications, or to do it on a soft surface like a couch. Here is where the nuance comes in: the data shows what is optimal for reducing SIDS, but there are many layers to safe sleep. Even if bed sharing or placing the baby on his or her tummy, there are viable ways to reduce risk.

I will end this section on a less somber note. Discussion about "safe sleep" is one of the most common conversations pediatricians have with parents of newborns and infants. My patients tend to be a little more "crunchy" than average and there are many parents that do speak to me about bed sharing. In general, I suspect the practice is more prevalent than most are willing to admit. Many of my parents describe experiencing special feelings of closeness with their child when they bed-share, such as love, bonding, and togetherness. These benefits are difficult to quantify and study, rendering the evaluation of their potential long-term benefits more challenging. Conversely, SIDS is an easy data point to study. We can see what people have and have not done in their homes when discussing SIDS outcomes and create guidelines around those data points. You can't really crunch data when it comes to quality of bonding. Or at least it is much harder. I understand the choices here are not easy, and even in light of the data, this decision is not cut-and-dry for many of you. My job is to inform you of the facts as we know them. You have to decide how to put them into practice for your family.

UNLOCKING THE MYSTERIES OF NEWBORN SLEEP

Newborns, bless 'em, are delightfully weird. Their underdeveloped systems lead to a lot of behaviors we would find straight-up worrisome in bigger kids (never mind adults)—and it's so hard to navigate what's normal and what's not when every little thing feels so important, both for short-term and long-term outcomes. Coming off the heavy topic of SIDS, for example, let me say I honestly believe one reason parents worry so much about it (besides it being our worst fear) is that newborn sleep itself is profoundly different from adult sleep and *it is weird*:

weird noises (what's up with the grunting?), weird movements (so much twitching!), weird breathing (*especially the breathing*). For the most part it is all normal, I promise!

Yeah, the breathing—there have been more than a few times I've been called by a frantic parent who told me their baby appeared like they stopped breathing for a few seconds while sleeping. "Stopped breathing"?! Normal. Seriously. Not a big deal (for the most part). How can this be? Well, newborns' brains are still working out how to correctly and consistently signal their bodies' systems. Because of this, irregular breathing is a pretty typical feature of newborn sleep. In the medical community, we call this "periodic breathing." (We need fancy words to justify the decade of medical schooling.) With periodic breathing, you might notice that your baby looks like they stop breathing for about five seconds, which is then preceded or followed by a burst of rapid breathing (fast, shallow breaths) for another five to ten seconds, after which they cycle back to regular breathing. This can happen numerous times during a sleep cycle, especially right after they first fall asleep. Periodic breathing is super common, especially in the first month, typically not a cause for concern, and usually stops around six months. (I hope the reason those monitoring devices can cause so much anxiety is now apparent to you.)

So, we've got freaky breathing to contend with, and then there are the sounds sleeping newborns make: gurgling, groaning, snorting, among other delightful noises. It's *loud* too. Surprisingly loud. We often hear people use the phrase "slept like a baby," but after having my own baby, I'm not sure that you really *want* to sleep like a baby. Again, for the most part, the odd noises are totally normal. Fun fact: newborns breathe mainly through their noses (and their airways are pretty narrow). This means even a tiny amount of mucus or dry air is going to result in noise. They also have much shorter sleep cycles than adults (about thirty minutes to an hour versus our more typical ninety minutes) and spend more of that in REM sleep (about 50 percent versus our 20 percent), also known as "active sleep." In other words, their sleep is more fitful—they have more frequent arousals and spend less time in deep sleep; they're going to stir, wiggle, and whimper. And because newborns eat off and on throughout the day and night, they are often digesting while sleeping; noises like grunting, burping, gurgling, and passing gas are par for the course. In general, if your baby is a noisy sleeper but otherwise seems fine, let them sleep. Don't try to reposition them or wake them up (unless you're a masochist). If they've pooped, sure, but do your best to keep the diaper change as unstimulating as possible: keep the lights low, keep quiet (now is not the time for narrating what you're doing). Nothing is wrong with your noisy sleeper—they're just being a newborn, living in a body that still hasn't upgraded to the latest software.

When it comes to monitoring your newborn's sleep, noisy breathing can be a concern that leaves many parents wondering when to seek medical advice. While some amount of irregular breathing is normal for infants, there are specific signs that should prompt immediate attention. These include pauses in breathing that last more than fifteen seconds, signs that your baby has stopped breathing and becomes limp, pale, or shows bluish coloration around the mouth. Additionally, if your baby's skin maintains a bluish tint even during periods of normal breathing, it's important to consult with a health-care provider. Last, rapid breathing should also be a cause for concern; in babies younger than six weeks, a rate faster than sixty breaths per minute is a red flag, and for those older than six weeks, a rate faster than forty-five breaths per minute warrants medical evaluation. These symptoms can indicate underlying issues that require prompt medical intervention.

In my experience, after parents learn that the symphony of sleep sounds their infant is capable of producing is normal and their anxiety around that topic dwindles, it's quickly replaced with a fixation on how much their newborn should sleep. Admittedly, that's often a focus right from the beginning—questions around sleep duration, total hours of sleep, daytime versus nighttime sleep, and the like, are among the most frequently asked questions I get. There's a lot to say here, but let's start with the very basics: newborns should be getting fourteen to seventeen hours of sleep in a twenty-four-hour period. The truth is, anything between the range of eleven to nineteen hours can be normal and healthy, depending on your baby. What most parents don't realize is that, in general, there are two kinds of newborns. There are those who sleep all the time (honestly, feeding is like a huge workout for them, so no surprise they're going to be tired a lot). Then there are those who are here to party—they just don't sleep as much and getting them down is definitely more of a challenge. Both are normal.

Even newborns who are awake more often, can, in general, remain awake only for so long. During the first three months of life, the average wake window for a baby is just sixty to ninety minutes. Then, typically, they'll sleep for a couple of hours before the next wake/sleep cycle starts again. In the first couple of weeks, it's unlikely they'll sleep longer than three or so hours at a time, as they'll wake to feed. Breast milk and formula are higher in sugar than fat, which is a brilliant design by nature—sugar digests more quickly than fat. This means newborns need to feed more frequently. Because their stomachs are so tiny, more-frequent feedings help them get the calories they need. In the rare case a newborn does sleep longer than two to three hours, you should generally wake them to feed in the first two weeks. The concern here is that while you might think they're getting enough food, they may not be, creating a vicious cycle in which they're sleeping longer because they're not getting enough calories. They don't have enough energy to be awake; they're lethargic, and the less time they're awake, the fewer calories they take in.

Once feeding is established, though—once baby is back to his or her birth weight, and baby's weight is going up (at about two weeks usually)—then if baby does happen to sleep a little bit longer, I tell parents, "you don't need to wake up baby. Just say thank you." Once you know that your baby is feeding well, gaining weight, and growing, it's less of a concern if he or she sleeps for more than a couple of hours. Some babies sleep for shorter stretches—even as short as thirty or forty-five minutes. As frustrating as this is, it's still within the bounds of normal. Sleeping longer than fifty minutes or so requires newborns to be able to connect their sleep cycles, which they may not be able to do, developmentally. They may rouse at the end of a cycle and not be able to soothe themselves back to sleep, as an adult would.

Bringing adult-based sleep expectations to newborns will leave you confused and likely frustrated. The biological mechanisms that tell us that nighttime is for sleeping—like the secretion of cortisol, the production of melatonin, and changes in body temperature—don't even begin to *emerge* in newborns until six weeks, and then not all at once. The natural body clock that helps us know when to wake up and sleep takes time to develop in babies. It usually takes about eighteen to twenty weeks, or around five months, for some babies to start sleeping through the night.

Given all this, it isn't helpful to think of a newborn's daytime sleep as "napping." I don't recommend parents put newborns on a schedule (and it is definitely not appropriate to attempt to sleep train a newborn; more on sleep training later on page 206). Every baby is going to be different.

They're not going to follow a schedule. You can dream, though. Whatever they do today is not necessarily going to be what they do tomorrow. Focus instead on just making sure they're getting some sleep and getting an appropriate amount of food.

In my opinion, it is far more important to be responsive to your baby's needs. Being mindful of your newborn's wake window (remembering it's only sixty to ninety minutes) and learning to check for their sleepy cues are among the best ways to help them establish a rhythm. Sleep cues in newborns include big yawns and rubbing their eyes and eyelids.

Inadvertently keeping a baby awake too long and overstimulating him or her can make it more difficult for the baby to fall asleep, leading to behaviors that can seem like colic (inconsolable crying, back arching, rigid posture). As your newborn's wake window draws toward its close, you'll want to start looking for sleep cues (and again, the length of the wake window can vary, so that's part of what you're learning here—it's a bit of a feedback loop in that sleep cues can signal the close of the wake window, but knowing the average wake window can remind you to look for sleep cues). Many parents do seem to believe that their newborns are awake more at night than during the day, supported by the accepted wisdom that newborns have day and night reversed (often explained as being a result of their time in utero, when mom's daytime motion lulled them to sleep). The daytime/nighttime switcheroo may just be an old wives' tale—it sounds truthy, sure, and many people swear by it and bring it up in office visits, but I have not seen any data to specifically support it. I do have one theory that is most definitely not backed by any data, but I'll tell you anyway. I think newborns are more awake at night because, from an evolutionary standpoint, this increased their chance of survival. Back in the day, if parents fell asleep at night, their baby wouldn't get the food it needed. By crying and being awake at night, babies kept their parents awake, ensuring the babies were fed every few hours. This additionally ensured that mom maintained an adequate supply of milk. Darwin at work here.

From a scientific standpoint, we are not interacting with and entertaining our little ones during their nighttime wake windows, so they are less tuckered out as a result. Moreover, milk supply tends to be lowest at night due to hormone shifts, which means babies may be getting just a little less milk and, therefore, are a little more hungry.

Many parents note that when they expect baby to be most tired—in the evening, after a long, stimulating day—baby, instead, is the fussiest and most difficult to soothe. Ahh, the "witching hour." No, it's not your imagination. Witching hour, usually defined as the period between 5:00 p.m. and 11:00 p.m., is a real thing. It tends to start up around two weeks and peak at six weeks. It's that time, every evening, just when *you* are at your most tired, that baby loses his or her shit. Nobody knows exactly why babies become fussier during this specific period (personally, my theory, and yes I always have a theory, is that it's really *parent* witching hour, when we're drained, exhausted, and less resilient, and this leads to a cycle of fussiness with our baby). Generally, the pervasive thought is that overstimulation and overtiredness are two of the major causes. If your newborn is super fussy and having a really hard time falling asleep, and you've ruled out any issues with their basic needs (i.e., are they hungry? Do they have a dirty diaper? Are they too hot or cold? Are they sick?), try some of the following to help soothe them:

- Swaddle baby to help them feel snug and secure (i.e., like they were in the womb).
- Go for a walk or car ride.

- Hold your baby in your arms, resting on their left side, to help with digestion, and gently rub their back.
- Walk your baby in a carrier, rock them, or try holding them in your arms while gently bouncing on a yoga ball.
- Offer your baby a pacifier if they'll take one—many babies are calmed by sucking.

The Baby Blues and Postpartum Depression

THE BABY BLUES

Even though I'm not an OB/GYN, an internist, or even a family medicine doctor, as a pediatrician, I'm one of the first (and often, only) doctors to see new parents—particularly new moms—in the days and weeks immediately following birth. In fact, most of the new moms I see don't even have their first scheduled OB/GYN postpartum checkup until six weeks after the birth of their child. From what I've heard firsthand, and from my own experience listening to my wife, the vibe of these postpartum appointments is mostly "has everything healed up/turned out okay?" In other words, the standard of care is based on an assumption that everything *has* gone well and is now status quo, despite all the possible complications women face in that initial month and a half postpartum. The ACOG revised its guidance in 2018 to recommend a checkup for postpartum patients at three weeks rather than six weeks. However, I can say, anecdotally, the six-week appointment is still the norm. It's as if once pregnancy is complete, the focus of healthcare providers switches entirely to the baby. Often moms are treated as if their health and well-being are no longer a priority, even though, in reality, the physical and emotional pain may be greater than it was during pregnancy.

This mindset is particularly dangerous to new mothers not only because of the physical complications that may follow birth, but due to the mental health issues that so prevalently accompany parenthood. As a pediatrician, I hold the very important privilege of checking in with new parents—especially moms—in those critical early weeks and days. Predominantly, I pay close attention to whether the mother and her partner (yes, as we will later touch upon, both partners can experience postpartum depression) are experiencing the baby blues or if those blues have persisted or deepened, which may signal the possibility of postpartum depression (PPD). Pediatricians are often the doctors who first screen for PPD, by attuning ourselves to your emotions. Parents may not know I am evaluating them for signs of PPD, scrutinizing the mood and emotions behind their responses and observing their interactions with me, each other, and the baby. If I am even slightly concerned, I will directly ask the parent or parents whether they are experiencing PPD. Some offices use written tools to screen for the baby blues.

Although this book is about babies and toddlers, self-care is an indispensable part of caring for your child. There is no parenting book without parents. Before we delve deeper into newborn wellness, I'm going to check in with *you*, just as I would if you visited my office. How are *you* doing? Parenting demands A LOT of you. One of the seemingly greatest benefits of parenting in the twenty-first century is the decreasing stigma and increasingly prevalent conversation around mental health and parenthood. If you don't feel totally blissed out after the birth of your baby, you are not alone. This is extremely common. The ensuing guilt engenders a shame spiral, further perpetuating the postpartum despair. It's truly a vicious cycle—hence the term "baby blues." Up to 80 percent of new parents experience them. Statistics don't lie: the baby blues do not discriminate. They can affect any parent, regardless of age, income, or education. No one "deserves" the baby blues and getting them doesn't mean you're doing something wrong.

Having the baby blues isn't just about experiencing feelings of sadness, though. They can also present as any of the following, alone or in combination:

- Feeling anxious, restless, and worrying more than usual
- Mood swings and crying "for no reason"
- Feelings of being trapped or a sense of regret
- Fear and guilt
- Irritability and grumpiness
- Difficulty focusing or concentrating
- Fatigue and insomnia

The baby blues usually kick in about two to three days after giving birth and last about two weeks, going away on their own without intervention. Although we are yet to pinpoint the exact cause of the baby blues, the general medical consensus is that they're likely the result of a combination of factors: the rapid postpartum drop in the hormones estrogen and progesterone, sleep deprivation, and the psychological and emotional experiences of giving birth and adjusting to life with a new baby. This is true for both first-time parents and parents who already have kids—in both instances, expectations may not align with reality, routines are upended, and family dynamics are deeply altered, all while you are expected to care for a helpless life that is completely dependent on you. No pressure, right?

The baby blues are normal and, frankly, to be expected. They don't require "treatment." There are, however, things you can and should do to lessen their impact on you.

- **Talk about it:** Talk to your partner, your friends, your family members, your doctors. Don't keep it to yourself.
- **Go outside:** I know—you haven't showered in days, there are questionable stains on your T-shirt, and no amount of deodorant will conquer that terrible body odor, but getting outdoors is critical for your mental health. Vitamin D—the "sunshine vitamin"—literally affects your mood and cognition. Just stretching your legs and breathing fresh air can make you feel less tired and trapped, and more resilient.
- **Eat well:** One thing I've noticed with a lot of new moms in my practice is that they're not eating regularly, because they're spending so much time caring for their baby, or they're not eating foods that support stable moods. Both a lack of calories and the "wrong" calories (i.e., lots of sugar and simple carbs) can cause "hanger" and energy crashes. Try to keep healthy snacks (fruit, pre-sliced veggies, hummus) near you.
- **Seek out support groups:** Many hospitals and birth centers run groups for new moms. There are also walking clubs, fitness groups, online groups, and classes specifically designed for new parents to attend with their babies.

Sometimes the baby blues persist, become more severe, or they were more severe in the first place. In such cases, you may need to consider the possibility that you are experiencing PPD.

POSTPARTUM DEPRESSION

The baby blues and PPD might appear similar at first, but with PPD, the symptoms are more intense and last longer. If untreated, PPD may render it more difficult, if not impossible, to care for yourself or your baby. PPD does not reflect on your fitness as a parent. It does not signify that you have done anything wrong. PPD is *not* a character flaw. No one deserves PPD or does anything to invite it. In my experience there inexplicably seems to be more self-imposed shame around PPD than the baby blues, and I suspect we can attribute this to the fact that people speak less openly about it. So many people don't realize how relatively common it is. Up to one in seven women, or 15 percent of women who give birth, experience PPD.

When it comes to navigating those early days of motherhood, it's essential to distinguish between the fleeting baby blues and the more serious PPD. The distinction lies in the duration of symptoms and the impact they have on your daily life. If those bluesy feelings persist beyond two weeks, you're likely moving into PPD territory, where emotions aren't just intense; they're relentless and disruptive.

For instance, while the baby blues might involve intermittent sadness, PPD often manifests as a more constant sense of despair. With PPD, anxiety can escalate into full-blown panic attacks and intrusive thoughts. Questioning your adequacy? That's common for new parents. With PPD, this morphs into an overwhelming sense of worthlessness and shame. While new parents are universally tired, PPD fatigue can feel like an insurmountable wall.

Symptoms might also include drastic mood swings, uncontrollable crying, or even thoughts of harming yourself or your baby. If you're experiencing the latter symptoms, seek urgent help. Call 911 or 988, the Suicide and Crisis Lifeline, immediately. You can also text HOME to 741741 to connect with a crisis counselor. This doesn't make you a bad parent; it means you're in a crisis that needs immediate attention. Seeking help actually makes you a good parent. If you're experiencing any symptoms of PPD, please talk to your doctor (primary care or OB/GYN) or speak to your child's pediatrician. We try to screen for it, and we can help you get the resources you need. Some parents feel I will judge them. They seemingly conflate their worth as a parent with a condition that is beyond their control when, in reality, some of the most excellent parents struggle with PPD. One has nothing to do with the other. I would never judge a parent struggling with PPD. I, and most pediatricians, want you to talk to us. We are here to help and support you and the baby. You simply need to open the door by saying something like, "Dr. Joel, I'm really having a tough time." There is no shame in this; in fact, it's just the opposite: acknowledging that something is wrong and seeking care is exactly what you *should* be doing. It is the very definition of *good* parenting.

Let's broaden the conversation about PPD to include the non-birthing parents, such as dads, partners, and even adoptive parents. Believe it or not, up to 10 percent of men may experience PPD after a new baby arrives. And guys, you're not immune to hormonal shifts either; levels of testosterone drop while prolactin, vasopressin, and oxytocin increase. The risk factors are pretty much the same as for women—stress, lack of sleep, a history of depression, and social pressures all contribute.

If your partner demonstrates signs, like irritability, a tendency to withdraw, or changes in sleep and eating patterns, don't dismiss these as trivial.

I've seen partners in my practice reluctant to admit they're struggling, fearing it makes them appear weak or feeling guilty about voicing their struggles when they perceive their partner to be bearing the brunt of the burden. Let's be clear: it's not a sign of weakness, and *your* emotional well-being is important too.

The same goes for adoptive parents or other caregivers. Introducing a new baby into the household changes its dynamics in ways that can be stressful for everyone involved. Nobody's emotional journey should be sidelined; after all, a healthy baby needs healthy caregivers all around. Parenthood, while challenging, should also offer moments of sheer joy. So let's ensure that every parent has the emotional support they need to fully engage in this life-changing experience.

Knowing what to watch for when it comes to PPD is one of the best ways to help someone struggling with it. Your partner is in a unique position to observe you, especially when your own judgment may be clouded. Remain amenable to difficult discussions, should the need for them arise. Getting help when it's needed could save your life—and your baby's.

Newborn Wellness

Physicians have been reciting the Hippocratic Oath for over *two thousand years,* solemnly pledging to heed the code of medical ethics that famously demands of them "First, do no harm" (okay, the actual translation is "I will do no harm or injustice to them [patients]," but it doesn't have quite the same ring to it, does it?). Nowhere in the oath does it say "I promise to keep my patients from ever getting sick." Why? Because we can't. That's not reality, and that's not our job as doctors. Many parents *do* seem to think this is *their* job, though. Allow me to disabuse you of this notion right now: it is not your job to keep your child healthy all the time. In reality, your job is to prepare your child's body, to the best of your ability, to handle everything that comes its way. You are not going to prevent your child from ever getting sick (unless you encapsulate your child in a bubble). You *can* help keep your child's body as healthy as possible, so when the next virus comes his or her way, your child has the best chance to fight it off easily and quickly.

Perfect health is not your goal (and not just because I'd be out of a job if this could be achieved). Still, parents come in often believing that a natural-minded lifestyle means their child *shouldn't* get sick. Some believe I possess the secret, magic elixir that combats all illness. Sadly, my medical license doesn't carry with it any supernatural powers. Even kids who lead the healthiest lifestyles get sick, especially when they start day care. It's unavoidable. Living healthfully doesn't grant you immunity superpowers. It *does* expedite the maturation of a newborn's still-developing physiological systems. Despite your best efforts, your kids will invariably come down with coughs and colds and upset stomachs. Newborns will spit up, experience diarrhea (just pray it's not while in their car seat), and make strange noises that seem more befitting of a demon than a cute baby. Your goal is overall long-term health, with the understanding that good health actually includes some mild sickness. That's just how the gluten-free, vegan, sprouted buckwheat cookie crumbles.

Understandably, many parents are afraid to let their child be sick. No parent wants his or her child to be uncomfortable. A parent may interpret discomfort as symptomatic of a more serious or worrisome condition. As a parent, I can attest to the fact that it is really, really difficult to watch your child feel bad, while you helplessly sit there, unable to make him or her better. Thus, we desperately scramble to do something—ANYTHING. Often, this results in your child's ingestion of a bevy of unnecessary medications and treatments that carry with them a corollary of avoidable side-effects—this, when in reality, time itself would likely heal the infirmity. This does not mean you should refrain from calling your doctor when your child is sick! *Please* call your doctor if something seems out of the ordinary. But not every gurgle is automatically reflux disease. Communicate clearly with your doctor, so your pediatrician can monitor your child's progress and determine if an illness has gone from mild to moderate or severe and if it requires medication. Newsflash: typically, time and love are the only remedies needed.

Even in newborns, most of the icky stuff doesn't require meds, just "watchful waiting." You may be frustrated when most of us pediatricians commonly mollify you with, "Wait it out. It will probably get better on its own." Thanks for nothing, doc, right? As a parent, you so badly want to allay your child's suffering and would happily surrender an essential organ to do so. As is true when you, yourself, are sick with a minor bug, medical intervention isn't imperative. You give your body time to heal. The same is true for children. If it's not super serious—as in *you-need-to-go-to-the-hospital-today*—then, in 99.9 percent of cases, you have the luxury to wait—to determine which direction things go. As a pediatrician, especially a more natural-minded one, I refrain from indiscriminately prescribing medication, when possible. I prefer to first track my patient's progress before committing my notoriously illegible doctor chicken scratch to prescription pad. In playing the waiting game, you give your child's body the necessary time to heal naturally. In the meantime, I educate parents on ways to naturally facilitate the body's healing. I prefer not to give medicine willy-nilly, except when there's an issue for which it is apparently medically required. If you have a pediatrician you trust (and that should be baseline), trust them.

CRYING AND COLIC

The bad news first: babies cry a lot. The good news: babies cry a lot and it's totally normal. In fact, during the first three months of life, babies cry, on average, *just over two hours a day*. In my experience, though, new parents don't anticipate just how much their baby will cry. A lot of parents come to me about crying (usually crying a little themselves . . . internally and externally). This is especially true when it comes to what they describe as inconsolable crying—their baby cried for twenty minutes nonstop and they couldn't soothe him or her. Their baby cried off and on all evening—*probably for at least an hour total!*—and it was very hard to calm them. Almost always NORMAL. There was even an instance where I received a frantic call from a mom about her six-week-old crying for about two hours. No other symptoms. Just out of character. On further questioning, she mentioned to me that they had just gotten home after an eight-hour drive, and mom was wondering if maybe that could have something to do with the crying fit. I calmly composed myself before replying, "Yes, yes. I do believe that may have something to do with it. I would probably be fussy for a few hours after an eight-hour drive as well." She laughed, I laughed. The tension diminished and she realized the question was a bit silly. While reading this story, you are probably thinking . . . well duh. But in the heat of the moment, after two hours of crying and zero hours of sleep, you may not be thinking straight. So remember, the crying is probably normal. But if you are worried, call the doctor.

Most parents who come to see me about their baby crying don't even come near to meeting the threshold for colic: three hours of crying (total, not necessarily in a row), three times a week, for three weeks in a row (otherwise known as "the rule of threes"), in an otherwise healthy baby. And, colic, while a huge blow to parents' quality of life, *is also normal.* Yes, we pediatricians have a general clinical definition of colic, but colic itself isn't a diagnosis of anything; it doesn't describe a pathology. Colic isn't a name for a disease or disorder—it's pretty much just a term we use for "crying a lot with no medical explanation." The fact that we need the term underscores how very commonplace colic is. In a sense, we have a name for a thing that doesn't exist, because this pattern of crying happens frequently enough that we needed a name to describe it.

There are different estimates for how many newborns are affected by colic, but most fall in the range of 20 percent, or one in five babies. It generally comes on in the second or third week of life, peaks at week six, and, for the majority of babies (60 percent), resolves by three months. By four months, colic resolves for 90 percent of babies. There aren't any identifiable "risk factors" for colic; it affects babies of both sexes equally and being breastfed or bottle fed hasn't been shown to make a difference. That's probably one of the most frustrating things about colic: it has no known cause. Yes, colicky babies do tend to be gassier and burp more, but most evidence has shown that is the result of swallowing air during crying episodes. Meanwhile, it's normal for all babies to be gassy. The most likely reason for their misery is just unfortunate human biology: our offspring, unlike most mammals, are born with immature nervous systems. For a newborn, merely existing can be uncomfortable and overstimulating. (It's Existentialist Philosophy 101.) The ability to self-soothe only improves as the nervous system matures.

Yes, colic-type crying *could* indicate other issues, such as reflux or gastroesophageal reflux disease (GERD), milk or protein allergies, illness, or injury—though only about 5 percent of cases of colic end up having an underlying cause found. If your baby seems like he or she is getting colicky, you'll want to look for any signs of illness, like fever or coughing; injury, like bruises; or discomfort, like a hair tourniquet (hair wrapped around a body part like a finger or toe). If your baby is crying inconsolably and has a fever, is vomiting, is lethargic, has diarrhea, or isn't gaining weight, he or she should be seen by a doctor right away. In any case, with severe and unusual crying, you should get your baby checked out. A doctor can not only check for the issues mentioned above, but also rule out things like hernia or corneal abrasions. Ultimately, you know your baby best. If your baby's crying becomes uncommonly frequent and lasts for an unusually long duration, he or she should be seen by a doctor. It doesn't have to be exactly three hours or for exactly three days or for exactly three weeks. The "rule of threes" is a frame of reference as opposed to a hard-and-fast law. You want to make sure you rule out any possible medical reasons and that, lucky you, your baby is "just" crying for no explainable medical reason: colic!

My bigger point here is that you should expect your baby to cry . . . like, a lot. Crying a lot does not constitute colic and it doesn't mean there's something wrong with your child (or with your parenting or caregiving) or that there is something for you to "fix." In fact, several studies have suggested that colic actually lies at the upper end of the normal range of crying for babies.

Colic itself isn't something you can "fix," either. Giving the pattern a name has had the unfortunate effect of equating it with an illness, which makes it seem like there should be a cure, or at least a treatment (there is some promising research around easing colic with probiotics, though—for a deeper dive on this, check out the section "Probiotics" in "A Wellness 'Medicine' Chest for Newborns" at the end of this section). Again, colic, though unpleasant for all, is normal. Ultimately, at its crux, colic is not the ostensible problem. *Rather, it is the way colic affects you and your family.* While most parents I encounter who have a colicky baby have expressed concerns over how colic will affect their child, there is no evidence to show that colic has long-term negative effects on children. Since colic got its official name back in 1954, there haven't been any studies I'm aware of that have shown it leads to harmful outcomes. Colicky babies grow into healthy toddlers and kids. For parents, coping with colic can be emotionally and physically taxing. It's really kind of cruel that colic kicks in right around week three to four—when you're deep in the throes of sleep deprivation. Your energy is at one of its lowest points. Your own tension and frustration make it difficult, if not impossible, to exude the calm necessary to soothe a screaming baby for hours, which ironically leads to a potentially worse cycle of crying.

The despondency is only exacerbated by the fact that we are hardwired to respond with urgency to our baby's cries. Being unable to soothe your baby for a prolonged period of time can and biologically does provoke anxiety, feelings of failure, panic, and extreme stress. You immediately enter that ignominious spiral, chastising yourself. You must be doing something wrong, right? All the babies on social media are so happy. As a minor, albeit significant, aside, I implore you to remember that what you see online is not reality. I take care of some fairly influential people, with some beautifully curated family social media feeds. Like seriously, they have millions of followers and you have seen their tabloid baby photos. I have backstage access to the wizard of Oz *behind* the curtain. Trust me when I tell you this formidable facade is in no way indicative of reality. I see the baby and family for their one-month visit; the mom is discombobulated and dishevelled. Later that very same day, mom posts a professionally taken photograph of the baby on social media. Beneath it, the caption reads: "Jade is 1 month old today. Our hearts are full. She could not be more perfect. Life could not be better. #blessed". This same mom just left my office lamenting about the rigors of parenthood, terrified there may be something wrong with her baby.

So many hide behind the proverbial curtain of social media, attempting to pass off fiction as reality. Don't drink the Kool-Aid. The difficulty of parenting a newborn is real and it's normal. You are normal. Your child is normal. Social media fantasy world is just that—a fantasy. And it is not normal.

If your baby does become colicky, the most important thing you can do for him or her is to take care of *yourself.* Like the preflight safety demonstration reminds us, put on your mask before putting on your child's. You're no good to your child if you, yourself, can't breathe. Coping with colic is really, really difficult. In the immediate moment of a bout of crying, you might feel overwhelmed. You may even feel angry. The best thing you can do for yourself and your baby in this moment is to set him or her down in a safe place (i.e., the crib) and step away. Take a deep breath and count to ten. In such scenarios, breathing exercises are generally helpful. Noise-canceling headphones are also helpful. Pop them on and set a timer for five minutes. This will not hurt your baby, I promise. In fact, the biggest danger to babies with colic are parents who are unable to manage their emotions and end up shaking them—so, please, take a break. At this point, do whatever will slow that heart rate down as quickly as possible. Maybe for you that looks like lying on the couch and visualizing a treasured place where you feel safe and happy. Maybe you get in ten minutes of exercise. Maybe it means relieving your sense of chaos by cleaning—sometimes a quick vacuum or running a loaded dishwasher just makes us feel in control, efficient, like *we've got this*, ya know? Or maybe it means calling a trusted friend or family member. Whatever you do, **remind yourself this will not last forever**. This is a phase. A crappy, unbelievably challenging one, but still only a phase. Remember, 90 percent of babies grow out of colic by four months. (Most families I work with seem much better just two weeks after I see their babies for suspected colic.) If you're still not feeling fully calm after ten or fifteen minutes, check on your baby, but don't pick them up until you've truly collected yourself. At that point, you can pick them up and run through your soothing techniques again.

In terms of the bigger picture of coping with colic, the most important thing you can do is get support for yourself. Don't be afraid to ask for help from friends and family. Tell your pediatrician. Consider joining a new parents group. I wish I didn't have to say this, but I do: in two-parent households, it is the job of *both* parents to care for their baby during episodes of crying, regardless of who is on leave or who is back at work. Take turns holding the baby. Refrain from blaming each other. Work as a team.

And give yourself grace—this is not your fault. Colic is not a reflection on you or your parenting or how your newborn feels about you. Your child will not end up on the therapist's couch, blaming your parenting for their colic. Our head goes there sometimes, though.

Reduce the expectations you typically place on yourself a little: this is not the time to hold yourself to the standards of your pre-baby life. Think of it as survival mode: you need to eat and sleep, and everything else is of lower priority. Let go of the idea that your house has to be clean. Outsource what you can if you're able to do so—this is a good time to try out one of the meal kit or grocery delivery services you've received 7,000 emails for. Limit your commitments and responsibilities to others beyond your immediate family as much as possible ("no" is a complete sentence)—focus on caring for yourself and your baby.

Seriously, the first two months or so are truly survival mode. You are meant to sleep. You have slept your whole life. Unless you did a medical residency, you probably didn't work a thirty-hour shift on fewer than five hours of sleep. Know that these first few months can be a little trying.

You may get a little tired . . . okay, REALLY tired. I get it. We all get it. I have been there. Remind yourself that it will get better. Much better. After colic, you have at least until their teen years before it gets that bad again.

GAS, GERD, AND BELLY PROBLEMS

Like clockwork, around one or two months, parents come to me to discuss the same ailment: GAS! Parents are very concerned about their gassy babies. Me, the doctor? Not so much. "But doc," I hear, "Liam is wiggling and fussing a lot. He pushes and strains so hard when he poops, his face turns red. And he's gassy at night *and* between feedings. What's wrong with him? He must have an allergy, right? I've eliminated (insert long list of delicious food items here) from my diet and switched formulas and he's still gassy!" Here's the thing, my friends: *every baby is gassy.*

To this day, I'm still not sure why people are so concerned with a baby's gassiness. In adulthood, we don't go around assuming that every fart is a sign of impending doom and disease (though, honestly, we grown-ups could stand to focus a little more on our gut health and a little less on our newborns' toots). Newborn babies, almost without exception, are gassy, fussy, wiggly, and not great at pushing out poop. My best guess as to why gas is such (generally unnecessary) cause for alarm is that as new parents, we're on high alert for something going on or being "wrong." Because of that persistent, low-grade worry, we're often *looking* for signs of illness—and gas is one of those things that is associated with lots of ailments, in the sense that, with pretty much any belly issue, there's going to be some gas. So, it's on the list for everything. A little reckless googling and you're down the gassy rabbit hole. But again, *every baby is gassy.* So, gassiness by itself doesn't really mean much.

From a medical standpoint, when a parent brings his or her baby in and expresses concern about gassiness, I check if baby is growing appropriately. Does baby appear lethargic and have difficulty waking up? Is baby feeding? Is he or she pooping and peeing? If everything else is status quo, a little bit of gas is generally not concerning. However, parents are very, very concerned about gas.

I blame it partially on the forums. More than one parent has explained to me that they read about a gastrointestinal issue on social media. (Dr. Joel angrily shakes his fist in the air at social media.) As Emily, a new mom to six-week-old Theo explained to me, "A lot of time, when I'm holding Theo while he naps, I'll scroll parenting groups on my phone and people are posting all of this stuff about their newborns having these very specific allergies and ailments. And I worry about what I'm missing. It's like, 'How do they know, how did they find out?' And then that makes me think, 'Oh, well, if Theo's making a gagging noise, he must have reflux disease.' All of these other parents I watched mentioned gagging and gas preceding their baby's diagnosis of GERD and one baby turned out to have a tumor. How do I know Theo doesn't have cancer?" It thus comes as no surprise that a generally innocuous symptom like gas can so easily lead us to a bad place.

How *did* those people on social media forums get those diagnoses? GERD, allergies, and other serious gastrointestinal issues must be as common as social media forums make us think, right? Wrong. Let's back up here for a minute. First—what is GERD? Well, the word itself is an acronym for "gastroesophageal reflux disease." Take away the "R" and you've got GER, "gastroesophageal reflux," otherwise commonly known as just reflux. Reflux happens when stomach contents come back up into a baby's esophagus and can present as regurgitation or spitting up. As a pediatrician in training, you learn quickly that almost all babies experience some degree of reflux—the sphincter muscle between the stomach and the esophagus isn't that strong in newborns and they spend a lot of time lying down, making it easier for fluids to flow from the stomach into the esophagus. In their first three months of life, about half of all babies spit up multiple times a day. Again, normal. Given all this, reflux on its own isn't a medical problem, per se. When it becomes more severe or chronic and leads to other symptoms, that's when it becomes GERD and requires treatment.

If you're concerned that your baby's reflux may have escalated to GERD, there are key signs to watch for. Red flags include poor weight gain, extreme fussiness after eating or throughout the day, forceful vomiting, frequent wheezing, fevers, severe back arching after eating, or blood in baby's stool. These symptoms suggest that it's time to seek professional medical advice to discuss GERD and other possible gastrointestinal concerns.

Basically, we're looking to see if the symptoms seem pathologic. This is where things get a little tricky because, when it comes to GERD, diagnosis is often an art as much as a science. In general, with GERD, a pediatrician is making a clinical diagnosis—one based on observed (as well as reported) signs and symptoms, rather than a diagnosis based on *testing*. We're considering how severe the presentation of reflux seems to be, which would then determine treatment or next steps, such as lifestyle changes, medications, or a referral for an upper GI endoscopy, a process in which a doctor inserts an endoscope (a flexible tube with a tiny camera at its end) into a baby's mouth and down to view their esophagus, stomach, and beginning of the small intestine, while also potentially collecting biopsies (small tissue samples) for further testing. Endoscopy is invasive and requires full sedation of a child. Most parents prefer to avoid it at all costs.

Notwithstanding the fact that most parents want to avoid endoscopy, they are also convinced that their baby's reflux is more severe than normal. Though some doctors will suggest lifestyle changes before initiating medication, in my experience (prior to opening my own practice), many doctors are quick to prescribe and many parents are unwilling to leave their pediatrician's office without a prescription in hand, such as for ranitidine or famotidine. There seems to be a "no harm, no foul" attitude vis-a-vis "trying" reflux medications. Consequently, reflux meds are overprescribed for newborns.

Let me give you an example from my practice. I'll never forget the parents who came to me for a second opinion just days before their four-month-old was set to undergo an upper endoscopy due to severe reflux and failure to thrive. The baby was on two reflux medications, but the prescriptions had done little to ease the reflux. The baby's doctor was recommending more invasive testing. I started by asking about the child's diet, making sure I had the full picture—was he breastfed? If so, had they ruled out any allergies to elements of the mother's diet? Formula fed? If so, what type of formula? *It turned out that diet had not even been touched on at the previous visit.* I learned that the parents had recently switched from breast milk to formula—and that, thinking back on it, the timing of the switch coincided with the onset of the severe reflux and failure to gain weight. The symptoms started around six weeks old, just a week or two after the introduction of formula. No one had put that together. The reflux, lack of weight gain, and pain only worsened over the next few weeks. The baby was placed on a medication and, when that didn't work, a second medication. No one was really thinking about the WHY. We agreed that before moving on to further testing the parents would try out a different type of formula for a few weeks and see if the reflux improved or even resolved. We adjusted the formula and miraculously (but not surprisingly) the symptoms improved significantly over the next month, so much so that the baby didn't need to go for the endoscopy. The reflux resolved, the parents avoided an uncomfortable and invasive procedure for their infant (not to mention the medical bills that would accompany it), and I gained a new family in my practice.

Let's take a moment to discuss Zantac, which at one time was dispensed to kids like candy. When I was in training, ranitidine (the generic name of Zantac) was the go-to medication for GERD. It was considered so safe that it was often prescribed at the mere mention of "bad reflux." On April 1, 2020, the Food and Drug Administration (FDA) issued an immediate withdrawal of all forms of ranitidine, including prescription and over-the-counter products, from the market, after findings that ranitidine products may contain unacceptable levels of a potential cancer-causing substance known as NDMA, or N-nitrosodimethylamine. This is one of those reminders that medications have side effects, some of which we may not learn about until subsequent research reveals them. The pros and cons of taking any medication should always be carefully weighed. Take a medication only if you really need it, because you never know what we may learn about a particular pharmaceutical a decade from now.

That is not to say medications are without value. However, recent studies have shown that 7 percent of infants are prescribed an acid inhibitor reflux medication. There has been a sevenfold increase in prescriptions over the last twenty years—despite their links to increased risks for infections and fractures in infants. It is additionally worth noting that, given the numerous studies showing these drugs' lack of efficacy in treating reflux in infants, the FDA has not approved them for use for children under a year old. The AAP has also recommended against their use in infants with GER—again, good old reflux—which appears to be the perfectly normal "condition" most of the children who take this medication have. In my practice, fewer than 1 percent of the babies I see ever need a reflux medication. I almost never prescribe it. The kids in my practice are not magical. We've simply adopted a different philosophy, one in which medications are a last resort. In my experience, in otherwise healthy children, reflux resolves on its own.

Despite what those internet forum people say, GERD is uncommon. Reflux is common and normal. The fact that a doctor says you *can* try a medication does not mean you should or *need* to. Many medications are overprescribed and, if you go into the doctor's office wanting a "quick fix," you will often leave with a prescription in hand. If instead you are armed with the knowledge that basically every parent comes to the one- or two-month well visit with a concern about gas and reflux (yet fewer than 1 percent actually require intervention), hopefully your concerns will be allayed. As parents, it's difficult to do nothing. We want to do something. That something may cause more harm than it seeks to prevent. Most of the time, doing nothing is the best thing you can do. Let your baby's highly intelligent body figure it out.

Yes, we should be attentive to our children's needs and attuned to anything outside their norm. At the same time, we must safeguard their health by not manufacturing problems that don't exist.

Poops and Pees

Welcome to the fascinating world of infant excretions! If you're a new parent, you'll soon discover that your baby's poop offers valuable insights into their health and well-being. Let's delve into the various aspects of infant stool, from the first meconium to the ever-changing frequency and what you can expect as they grow.

Frequency: Though the frequency with which a baby poops varies from kid to kid (just like with adults), you can expect your little one to have his or her first poop within twenty-four hours of birth (many hospitals won't release a baby who hasn't passed their first bowel movement). This first poop is called meconium. It's typically dark green, almost blackish, tar-like, and sticky. Fun fact: meconium is formed by your baby swallowing amniotic fluid (and all the stuff it contains, like skin cells and hair) in the womb. Your baby's intestines absorb the water in the amniotic fluid, and the remaining substance—the meconium—lines the large intestine. By the time a baby is full term, their intestines are filled with meconium. Pooping this out after birth is a great sign that baby's digestive system is functioning as it should.

Occasionally, a baby will pass meconium before they're born (this mostly happens in babies who have gone past forty weeks). Normally, this is not a big deal. It's a little icky to think about, but swallowing meconium won't harm your baby. If your baby inhales meconium, though, that's another issue. Because meconium is so thick and sticky, aspirating it can make it hard to breathe and cause respiratory distress. Amniotic fluid that has meconium in it is pretty hard to miss—it's usually greenish in color—and doctors and nurses are trained to look for it. If they spot it, they'll check your baby for signs of distress (such as a blue tinge to the skin, nostril flaring, grunting, or a change in heart rate). If your baby is active and crying, there's nothing to worry about.

After they've passed the meconium, the rate at which any given baby poops is pretty variable. In my experience, this is one of those things that really surprises parents and often causes unnecessary alarm. In the first week of life, some babies have a bowel movement after every feeding. Some babies poop once a day. Whether a baby is breastfed or formula-fed also affects frequency—the former tends to poop more often than the latter because breast milk is more easily digestible and passes through the digestive system more quickly.

After the first two or three weeks, the frequency with which a baby poops really slows down. At this point, it can be normal for a breastfed baby to go without pooping for up to a week (though I wouldn't say once a week is ideal)! Just be prepared with *a lot* of wipes, if this is the case. As long as your baby is nursing regularly, gaining weight appropriately, and his or her stools are soft, your baby's good—in other words, going a few days without pooping is not necessarily a sign of constipation. If it's been more than three to five days and your baby hasn't pooped, then it's time to pick up the phone and check in with your pediatrician. If your baby is formula-fed, he or she should poop at least once every couple of days. Don't be shocked if the stooling frequency changes as your child gets older. He or she may usually poop every day, then all of a sudden go two days without one, then have a big poop and go back to every day. This is very normal. The bottom line for both is this: it's good to have a sense of how often, in general, your baby poops, but as long as your baby is feeding normally and gaining weight, you don't need to stress about his or her exact number of poops and you don't need to worry if it has been a day or two without a poop.

Color and Consistency: After the first couple days, babies should have passed all their meconium. After this point, if baby's poops are still looking very dark green or black, check in with your pediatrician. Typically, though, around day three, babies start producing "transitional poop." For both breastfed and formula-fed infants, these stools are yellowish in color. Both will have very soft, almost runny stools at this point, but a breastfed baby's will be more "seedy," almost like it's flecked with sesame seeds.

Around day five, babies start producing regular old poop. If your baby is breastfed, you can expect their poop to continue to be seedy, soft and mushy, or loose and liquidy, mixed with more solid particles. Their poop will be mustard colored (though if the breastfeeding parent is eating a lot of greens, you might see a greenish tinge to the poop) and typically not very stinky. If your baby is formula-fed, their poop will be firmer and more like paste, but in general no more so than peanut butter, and might be on the stinkier side. You can expect your baby's poop to be lighter yellow or tannish. It's normal for both breastfed and formula-fed babies to have a bit of mucus in their poop. It's worth noting that just because formula-fed babies have poop with different characteristics, it doesn't mean formula is bad. Each type of feeding has its own set of nutritional components that affect bowel movements, and neither is inherently negative. There is going to be a lot of crossover in terms of the appearance or consistency.

Once you introduce solids to a baby's diet at around six months, those diapers will start to look and smell quite different. Your baby's poops will get firmer, and a lot more green and brown (or other colors . . . let's just say you'll know if your little one had blueberries or beets for lunch). If you're doing baby-led weaning (see page 152) and baby is eating finger foods in addition to or in place of purees, you'll probably see undigested bits of food in there (like the skins of fruits and vegetables). Due to the extra fats and (natural) sugars in their diet, the odor of their poop will also become much stronger. Fun fact: If you feed your baby bananas and they poop frequently, they may have poop that looks like it contains worms. It's not worms, it's just the undigested banana strings.

What to Watch Out For: Before the introduction of solids, the color of a baby's poop will generally fall along that yellow-tan-brown spectrum (just like a 1970s den). Other colors, such as white or red poops, could be cause for concern and are worth a call to your pediatrician. White or very pale poops are generally still normal but are a reason to get checked if persistent (though they may follow a stomach bug or certain medications). If you see red *in* your newborn's stool, that may be blood and also warrants follow-up. There are three things to keep in mind here: one, newborn girls may have a "mini-period" after birth, as they process hormones absorbed in utero from their mom—you may see a couple of drops of blood in their diaper or on their poop, which is normal; two, if your baby has a diaper rash with some minor irritation around the anus, you might also see a little blood on the surface of his or her poop; three, if you see a reddish tinge in a newborn diaper that also has some urine, it is likely urate crystal, which is normal in the first week (more on that in "Urination").

If your baby's poops are hard or very dry and they're *really* struggling to get them out, that—along with going longer than three to five days consistently—is a sign of constipation. In most cases, constipation is diet-related.

Also warranting mention are the variety of sounds, movements, and expressions newborns tend to make while pooping, such as grunting, wiggling, straining, turning red, grimacing, and exhibiting an astounding range of other facial expressions. As long as their stools are soft, this is not a sign of constipation. Their stomach muscles are not super strong yet, and on top of that they are less than skilled at using them to apply pressure while also relaxing their pelvic floor (that's how us talented grown-ups do it . . . or should). It's hard work for them to coordinate all these functions!

Last, but not least, we have good old-fashioned diarrhea: multiple very loose, very watery stools a day. Diarrhea is among the top reasons to be grateful for modern medicine. Before the twentieth century, many of the (now-eradicated or well-controlled) diseases that accounted for the high rates of childhood mortality worked their insidious damage primarily via causing diarrhea. Diarrhea can be very dangerous for newborns because of how quickly it leads to dehydration, but it can also be hard to spot, given that newborns already have very soft and runny poops. For all babies, the telltale sign of diarrhea *is a sudden increase in frequency of poops.* If this lasts for three or more poops, it's likely diarrhea. Coupled with that, if there is *a lot* of mucus in the poop and it smells especially bad, it's likely diarrhea. Other clues, alongside the suspect poop, would be less interest in feeding and fever.

Diarrhea is considered "mild" when there are three to five watery stools within twenty-four hours; "moderate" when there are six to nine watery stools within twenty-four hours; and "severe" when there are ten or more watery stools within twenty-four hours. You should call your doctor right away if your baby has diarrhea and you suspect dehydration; if they're less than a month old and have mild or moderate diarrhea; and at any age if they have severe diarrhea.

URINATION

Frequency: While I wrote almost a micro novella on baby poop, there's just not as much to say about pee. It's a lot simpler. All your newborn does is drink, and breast milk and formula primarily consist of water. There is not as much variety or excitement to be had in terms of frequency, color, or consistency. As a matter of fact, for baby's first week (up to day seven), we even have a rule of thumb when it comes to how often he or she should pee: generally speaking, it's at least one wet diaper per day of life. To break it down for those who prefer a tidy list, that's:

- One wet diaper on day one (first twenty-four hours)
- Two wet diapers on day two
- Three wet diapers on day three

You get the idea.

See, like I said, not complicated, right? After that, it's normal for a baby to pee at least six times a day, but some pee as often as every three hours (a newborn's tiny bladder can hold only about a tablespoon of urine), kind of like me after some coffee.

When they're ill, have a fever, or the weather is super hot, a baby's usual output of urine (or wet diapers) can drop by as much as half. In order to know when to be concerned, you need to know what's normal for your baby in the first place. For that reason and others, tracking your baby's wet diapers, both in that first week and after, is, in my opinion, a little more useful than keeping a meticulous ledger of their bowel movements. When you track wet diapers, you're also tracking how well they're feeding and feeling. For example, if your baby goes from four wet diapers to ten, that could alert you that he or she might have a UTI. If your baby usually has nine wet diapers a day and suddenly starts having only two, this might signal that he or she may not be getting enough fluid or may be losing too much. For breastfeeding moms, this can be especially helpful, as it's hard to know just how much milk a baby is consuming. You probably don't need to jot down every time your baby pees. However, it's good to keep in mind a general frame of reference and be on the lookout for major swings in frequency.

What to Watch Out For: After the first week, if your baby has fewer than four wet diapers a day, or goes more than eight to ten hours without a pee, call your pediatrician.

Red, orange, or brown pee could indicate blood in the urine. Regardless of whether your baby is a boy or a girl, after the first week, this would not be normal. Blood in urine could reveal any number of serious issues like infection, kidney stones, or a compromised immune system, among others—so you should see your pediatrician ASAP. Similarly, cloudy pee—especially if it's accompanied by a color change—requires a call to the doctor, as it could signify a UTI or kidney infection.

Finally, there's strong smelling pee—and I don't just mean stinky pee. If baby is a little dehydrated (clue: baby's pee will also be on the darker side), it is normal for his or her pee to possess an odor. This should resolve with the intake of more fluids. In contrast, really malodorous pee can indicate a bacterial infection.

THE GREAT DIAPER DEBATE

Now that we've explored the contents of your child's diapers, let's shift our focus to the diaper itself. Whether it's cloth or disposable, each type comes with its own set of pros and cons. I wish I could say I'm surprised that there are some who are very militant about the "right" kind of diapers to use. Alas, we live in such a tribalized moment that I would be far more surprised if there was a consensus on the subject. Yes, I'm talking about cloth versus disposable diapers. Here's a surprise for ya: I am not opposed to disposable diapers.

Cloth diapers are practically one of the "ten commandments" of crunchy parenting. They're indisputably better for the environment. Disposable diapers are seen as "easy" and for some twisted reason we equate difficulty with virtue. I am here to tell you that doing things the hard way is not *inherently* better than opting for convenience. Choosing the hard way is not an automatic reflection of your moral or ethical uprightness—though it's treated that way, especially by some of the more extreme members of the natural-minded community.

You gotta do what you gotta do. You shouldn't feel bad about using disposable diapers if that's where you're at. I do, however, have a strong opinion on "luxury" diapers that seem to be popping up everywhere these days. Luxury diapers! I feel like I lost a few brain cells just typing that. In general, these seem like just another unnecessary way to separate parents from their income. Terming them "luxury" does not render them devoid of harmful ingredients, either. When you're bombarded with targeted ads extolling their virtues, it's easy to doubt yourself.

When it comes to what to worry about with diapers, the more important choice to me is being mindful of what you put on your kiddo's body. Diapers are in contact with your baby's skin nearly 24/7 for at least two years. It's easy to forget (but I will remind you) that skin is an organ.

Most disposable diapers work so well at absorbing pee and preventing leaks because they're full of superabsorbent polymers (SAPs) like sodium polyacrylate, which can absorb over three hundred times its weight in water. That might sound scary, but there's been a lot of testing of SAPs. There is very little evidence that they're harmful—and fortunately, they are generally locked away inside the core of disposable diapers.

What's more concerning are the chemicals we *know* may be harmful and that *are* frequently found on the outer layer of diapers, sometimes called the top sheet, which sits directly against baby's skin. The problem is, since diapers are considered a consumer product rather than a "medical device," they're regulated by the Consumer Product Safety Commission (CPSC), rather than the FDA. The CPSC doesn't require diaper companies to reveal what's in their diapers or to test them for safety (with the exception of lead testing).

Given this, if you are going to use disposable diapers, I'd encourage you to only buy brands that do disclose what goes into their diapers, or at minimum, that are explicit about what is *not* in their diapers. Look for diapers that limit their use of plastic components and are free of these biggies: **chlorine, dyes, fragrances,** and **phthalates**.

(And if you were wondering, we used disposable bamboo diapers on Eli.)

Body Care

DIAPER RASH

Allow me to remind you of the obvious: babies sit around in their own pee and poop. No matter how fastidious you are about changing your baby's diaper, diaper rash is inevitable. Prolonged contact with moisture breaks down the skin, causing not only irritation, but also greater susceptibility to bacteria (now, what naturally occurring substance produced in large quantities by babies might be full of bacteria? hmm . . .). In addition, the same design and materials that make diapers leakproof also prevent air-flow. Combine *that* with chafing and rubbing, and it's kind of astonishing that babies don't have diaper rash all the time.

Diaper rash is super common. Approximately half of all babies will develop diaper rash at some time (though, anecdotally, I have not seen a baby in my office that *never* had diaper rash). Technically, there are several different kinds of diaper rash, but since the reality is that they all cause similar discomfort for your little one, the bigger issues are preventing them, treating them, and knowing when it's time to see a doctor.

The single most effective weapon against diaper rash is changing your baby's bottom frequently. Nobody loves diaper changes (including baby), and diapers don't come cheap, but dry skin equals fewer rashes. Ideally, you want to change your baby right after every poop or pee. The reality is you aren't going to always know right away, and, generally, you aren't going to wake a sleeping baby.

Next, keep in mind how delicate a baby's skin is. Don't rub! Patting and gentle wipes are all that's required. Rubbing at your baby's skin can damage its moisture barrier and irritate it, priming it for diaper rash. If the mess is particularly bad, you can drape a wipe over the area and give it a minute to dampen the situation, making it easier to wipe away. Speaking of wipes, choose wipes that are alcohol and fragrance free to further cut down on the possibility of irritating the skin. You can also use a squirt bottle filled with warm water and gently rinse your baby's butt, or soak his or her tushy in warm water. By this, I mean you can basically make your own baby bidet. (Sidenote . . . if you don't have a bidet for yourself, I highly recommended one. You'll thank me later.)

You may also use a soft cloth and a non-soap cleanser for cleanup. Whatever you choose, make sure your baby's tush is dry before you put that diaper back on. We're talking arid, Joshua Tree in August kind of dry. To get there, pat; don't rub. Or you could do Eli's favorite: the diaper fan. Just wave that diaper back and forth like your baby is an emperor and you're one of his minions (because you essentially are), fanning him with a giant palm leaf. Finally, I've known some parents who are not above simply blowing on their kids' rear ends.

Before you seal up that diaper, ice that tushy like a cake . . . with diaper cream, of course. Thought diaper cream is only for treating rashes? Wrong—it's really, really great at preventing them, because it creates a barrier between the skin and all the moist icky stuff. Be generous with it.

This is not the time for moderation. There's no such thing as too much butt cream. There are many types of diaper cream. For general everyday moisturizing, I like to go as natural as possible. Avoid the chemicals. I'm talking some serious woo-woo here like calendula, aloe, lavender, jojoba, shea. If you are seeing some of these words on the label, you are in the right place. For severe rashes, think more of a barrier cream. Barrier diaper creams generally contain either zinc or petrolatum. I am a fan of the zinc-based creams, but I imagine you guessed that by now.

Allowing your baby to chill with no diaper is also great for preventing (and treating) diaper rash. Circulating air helps tame moisture and forgoing a diaper also prevents moisture from becoming trapped in the first place. Tummy time is great for this. Just place a towel underneath your baby to absorb any accidents and make sure it's a comfortable temperature in the room.

When securing any diaper, be certain you're not pulling it closed too tightly (and that your baby is wearing the right size diaper). It may feel satisfying to *you* to stretch those tabs as far as they will reach across baby's tummy, but tight diapers create chafing, which can cause or worsen diaper rash. Obviously, you want the diaper to fit well, but it doesn't need to be secured like Fort Knox.

As much as you may think I love writing about infants' bodily waste and how to secure it optimally, I really don't. Like you, I'm only human. That's why I'm relieved to say that the best way to treat diaper rash is . . . to do all the same things you would to prevent it.

The real question is, how do you know when diaper rash has crossed from nuisance territory into health concern? Call your pediatrician when:

- The rash does not improve, or gets worse, after a few days of home remedies.

- The rash is crusty, includes sores, blisters, or pimples, or the skin is peeling where the rash is or around it.
- The rash is so painful to baby it's difficult to treat, or to clean baby up.
- Baby develops a fever along with the rash.
- Baby is taking antibiotics and develops a very red or bright pink rash with clear edges that may or may not have little bumps along them (this could be a sign of a yeast infection).

It's worth keeping in mind that if you are changing baby frequently, being gentle with cleaning, using diaper cream, giving them naked time, and so on, and he or she still keeps getting frequent diaper rashes or baby has a diaper rash that won't go away—but isn't the result of a yeast or a bacterial infection (as per your doctor)—your baby might just be allergic to the brand of diapers you're using, or to one of the other care products such as the wipes or cream. The dyes, elastics, fragrances, and preservatives used in diapers, wipes, and creams are common allergens. Trying a new brand of each (one at a time) for two weeks can help you figure out if one of these may be the culprit.

UMBILICAL CARE

Dealing with the umbilical cord stump is surprisingly intimidating and a common source of anxiety for many of my new parents. The funny thing is, there really isn't much to do. The basic rule of thumb is: LEAVE IT ALONE.

In general, you can expect the cord stump to fall off when baby is about two weeks old. It *can* come off in less than a week and it *can* take up to a month or a bit longer—but those are the far ends of the "normal" spectrum. In the meanwhile, the stump is going to be a little gross. There's no getting around that. It can be kind of scabby and oozy as the wound beneath heals. As the stump dries out, it goes from yellow to dark brown or black. It might stink a little. It's normal for there to be a few spots of blood.

During this time, you want to keep the stump dry. Sponge baths only during this period, and try to give your baby some naked time or diaper time where the stump is exposed to air.

Some natural-minded parents do ask about applying goldenseal powder to it. Goldenseal is an herb in the buttercup family, native to North America. Its root contains berberine, which may have antibacterial effects. While I've not personally seen any issues crop up with its use in my practice, it is not recommended by the AAP. If you wish to use goldenseal powder, you should always check with your pediatrician before doing so (and be aware that it stains).

Once the cord falls off, there might be a little bleeding or a little drainage of fluid, especially on the earlier end of the spectrum. If you notice a lot of blood or pus, you should get baby checked out. Contact your pediatrician if there is spreading redness around the stump or it is hot to the touch. Once the stump falls off, you can go ahead and give your baby their first "real" bath within a few days.

Congestion, Gagging, and Hiccups

From sniffles to hiccups, it may seem like your newborn is tackling a symphony of bodily noises and functions! While it's tempting to sound the alarm, most of these little quirks are usually no reason for concern. I was tempted to title this section "The Symphony of Normalcy" because, aside from illness in newborns, these common occurrences are rarely anything to fret about. They may not win any beauty contests, but they're a regular part of newborn life.

Congestion: Nasal congestion in particular is one of those things that, again, is *very* common in newborns. Their nasal passageways are so small (just two to three millimeters wide) that it's normal for mucus to collect in there—particularly when they are lying down—leading to noisy breathing. Parents often identify this as congestion. In the first month or first couple months, it's super common for parents to report to me—with worry—that their kid is a noisy breather or that they're "congested a lot." The baby will be totally fine otherwise—happy, smiling, eating normally, no fevers—but the parent hears a noise every now and again. It's just mucus in there. Newborns make a lot of mucus in response to the smallest irritation or any inflammation, especially if they have a mild cold. Babies who aspirated a little meconium at birth, but who are otherwise healthy and doing fine, might still be producing some extra mucus the first few days. Smoky air, pollutants, viruses, and weather changes can all cause an uptick in your little one's productivity as a snot factory. In general, snot is a good thing for babies—it keeps the mucous membranes lining their nose lubricated (making it *less* irritating to breathe) and filters dust and dirt from their lungs.

If you feel that your baby is so stuffed up they're uncomfortable or having trouble sleeping or feeding easily, you can use a suction bulb to try to clear their nose a bit. Just don't overdo it; babies *need* a little mucus to keep their airways healthy. To use a bulb effectively, squeeze the bulb (preferably not right in your baby's face) and then, still squeezing, gently insert the tip of it in baby's nose. Seriously, you only need to insert the tip. Release your grip to suck out the snot. Satisfying! Squeeze out the goo in a burp cloth or whatever you have handy and rinse the bulb by squeezing and releasing it a few times in clean water. Repeat on the other side. Et voila! (If you're feeling brave, you can try one of those tube-style snot suckers that requires *you* to do the sucking.) And, please, if your baby really doesn't like having mucus forcibly vacuumed out of his or her airways (sounds fun, right?)—if your baby's crying and freaking out—give the little guy or gal a break. Your baby's nasal passageways are probably irritated, tender, or sore, and poking around in there is not going to give him or her enough relief to make it worth it.

Sometimes parents report that their child has chest congestion. It's more than likely that what they're hearing is mucus in the nasal passages. Babies' bodies are small and it can be difficult to distinguish where breathing sounds originate because of this. Parents will sometimes describe congestion noises as "wheezing." Wheezing is a serious concern when it comes to breathing. Typically, wheezing is a high-pitched whistling sound produced when a baby exhales and is heard while listening with a stethoscope. Wheezing is caused by a narrowing of passageways in your baby's lungs. It can be hard to distinguish "true" wheezing from other similar noises if you're not a doctor (especially without a stethoscope). If you're worried about your baby's breathing, always get him or her checked out. Taking a video for your doctor may also be helpful.

Bottom line, if your baby is having difficulty breathing, having trouble getting in air, flaring his or her nostrils when breathing, breathing really fast (where their belly is going in and out hard and fast; typically more than forty breaths per minute), or turning blue in the face (especially around the lips or nostrils), take him or her to be seen immediately.

Mostly, when parents come in concerned about nasal congestion and the resultant noisy breathing, it's usually normal. If a baby is happy, alert, feeding well, and not sick, congestion is not a problem.

Gagging and Hiccups: Babies are born with the gag reflex—and this reflex is pretty freaking awesome. It might not *sound* awesome—it might, in fact, sound horrible—but it can be literally lifesaving, designed to help protect unfamiliar objects from entering the lungs. At birth, the gag reflex is fairly sensitive: triggering it begins closer to the front of the mouth. As babies get older, it moves farther back (otherwise, we'd never be able to learn to eat solid food). For brand-new babies, gagging can happen in response to a bit of fluid in the mouth. In utero, babies' lungs are filled with fluid; during labor, their bodies produce chemicals that help them expel this fluid. In the case of a vaginal delivery, the pressure and force of birth pushes out most of what remains. It's not unusual for a little bit of fluid to be left behind. In the first couple of days of life, a newborn might cough to expel it. The fluid can collect at the back of the throat, causing gagging. Thereafter, it's normal for newborns to gag occasionally. Newborns might typically gag a little during or after feeding (if breastfeeding, this might be due to a strong letdown and if bottle feeding, this might be a result of using a nipple with too fast a flow), or as a result of reflux.

Speaking of reflexes, hiccups start in utero. While I can't speak to the sensation itself, I do remember when my wife, Sarah, first started feeling our son's hiccups in her second trimester. It was so funny realizing that Eli was in there, already experiencing one of life's great mysteries: *Why do we hiccup?* Nobody knows. The mechanics of hiccups are pretty straightforward: the diaphragm spasms, causing a change in pressure in the throat, which in turn causes the vocal cords to clamp, creating the "hic" sound. Why our brains signal us to hiccup is another matter. Just like occasional hiccupping in an adult is normal, so are occasional hiccups in a baby.

The main takeaway here for parents is that you don't need to be worried about a random cough or sneeze, hiccupping now and then, the infrequent gag, or intermittent "noisy breathing" (congestion). If something is consistent or getting worse, or you're worried, get it checked. Breathing is a big deal and should be taken seriously. Just don't let every little noise send you into a panic.

When to Worry About a Newborn

I admit it: when it comes to new parents, "You don't need to worry too much about . . ." has practically become a mantra for me. Admittedly, there *are* times when an easy-breezy, laid-back attitude isn't gonna cut it. Your five-year-old has a slight fever? Meh. Your newborn has a fever? BIG DEAL.

In general, in the first month or two of life, babies face more challenges from the very same illnesses or injuries we would consider a nonevent in older kids. We doctors worry about newborns a lot more. They're just more susceptible to serious outcomes. If you're extremely worried, trust your intuition. If you're so worried that you are contacting me at 2:00 a.m., I'm worried, because I trust your gut instinct as a parent.

Unfortunately, I'm not with you when your child starts vomiting on the family vacation you've been looking forward to for the last three months. I can't tell you whether or not this is one of those "oh crap" moments or more of an "Order *Moana* from Pay-Per-View, call in some room service for yourself, and let your kid rest" moments.

Even though I can't tell you definitively whether to cancel your reservations and head for the ER, I can walk you through the signposts I look for when I assess the severity of a patient's condition. Please note, though, this is far from an exhaustive list of every sign or symptom that *could* signify a serious condition requiring immediate medical attention; these are merely a few of the most common issues that cause me concern.

Fever: Anytime a newborn has a temperature that's over 100.4 degrees, it's a big deal. In a baby under a month old, you will almost always need to go to the emergency room for a full work-up. Between ages one and two months, you will always need to bring your baby to be seen and evaluated by a doctor, and, still, your baby will often need to go to the ER.

Trouble breathing: I don't mean your baby has a stuffy nose or is congested. If your baby is struggling to take in breaths, if you see any retracting while breathing (the chest pulling in at the ribs, below the breastbone, or above the collarbones), if your baby is breathing rapidly (more than sixty breaths a minute), or if his or her nostrils are flaring every time he or she inhales, your baby should be seen.

Lethargy: This term has a very specific meaning in the context of medicine, so use it wisely with your pediatrician. Babies sleep a lot. Being sleepy in and of itself is not usually a concern. When *awake,* your child should be alert. If your baby is not alert, if he or she stares into space and does not respond to you, if he or she is much less active than usual, if you find it difficult to wake up baby from sleep, or if baby is not showing interest in feeding, and he or she is getting progressively more floppy and less responsive due to illness, dehydration, exhaustion, *that's* lethargy—and your baby needs to be seen *immediately.*

Dehydration: Anytime your newborn shows signs of dehydration, such as decreased urine output or dry lips, no matter how seemingly "mild," you should check in with the doctor. If your baby is showing any signs of severe dehydration, including significantly decreased urine output, sunken fontanelle, very dry and cracked lips, and no tears, he or she needs to be taken to an ER right away. Untreated dehydration could lead to seizures, heatstroke, and even organ failure.

Trauma: Unfortunately, I don't know one parent who hasn't accidentally dropped his or her baby or whose baby hasn't experienced an accidental fall (rolling off the bed, couch, or chair seems to be the most common scenario). This is the reason we opted for cork floors in our living room. Most days of the week, Eli's head thanks us. Always stay vigilant when you place your baby on any surface, but don't beat yourself up when (not if) it happens to you. Babies are surprisingly tough and resilient—they're almost always fine after a fall. That said, any major trauma, especially alongside other symptoms such as vomiting or loss of consciousness, justifies an exam right away. With any drop or fall from a large height, we should have a look.

The tricky issue with head injuries is that there is no easy or obvious way to know what's going on inside the brain. When parents message me about an injury that involves hitting the head, it's often difficult to advise. The big concern is that your child landed in such a way or hit his or her head with enough force to cause internal bleeding. That's what us physicians are attempting to ascertain—what kind of fall was it? Theoretically, a minor fall could cause such an injury. It's far less likely, though—especially if the fall is from less than a foot or onto carpeting. A good rule of thumb is, if you're worried, call your doctor. Don't worry about worrying too much. The questions a doctor is likely to ask you, and which are worth considering yourself, are meant to assess severity: does baby have a huge goose egg or a small knot (or no bump at all)? Has he or she thrown up? Do your baby's eyes look normal? Is he or she able to focus and track movement?

If your doctor has you head for the ER, or you choose to go there yourself, the ER doctors will likely employ the Pediatric Emergency Care Applied Research Network Head Injury Decision Rules (PECARN Rules) to determine if your child needs a CT scan. It remains a very mainstream position in pediatrics that, in order to limit a child's exposure to radiation, CT scans should be avoided unless necessary. The PECARN Rules, which take into account the child's age, level of consciousness and symptoms, have been hugely successful in identifying potential traumatic brain injuries in young children, while greatly reducing CT usage.

The good news, though, is that 97 percent of the time, falls are not serious—they might leave a bruise or a bump, but they won't do lasting damage.

A WELLNESS "MEDICINE" CHEST FOR NEWBORNS: NATURAL REMEDIES AND SUPPLEMENTS

Babies under two months can't take and should never be given over-the-counter medicines such as Tylenol or Motrin (remember, if your baby has a fever of 100.4 degrees or higher, they need to be seen by a doctor *immediately*). That said, there are some natural remedies and supplements that might be appropriate for the newborn crowd that parents can keep on hand in their home wellness cabinet. The following are the ones I recommend most, but it goes without saying that *before* starting any form of supplementation or giving your baby any new remedy, you should *always*, without exception, speak to your pediatrician first, to make sure the dosing and form is appropriate for your baby's age and personal situation.

Vitamin D

Adequate vitamin D, also known as "the sunshine vitamin," is critical for our health: it helps our bodies absorb calcium and phosphorus, both of which are crucial for bone density; prevents rickets in children; helps bolster the immune system; regulates blood sugar; helps safeguard cardiovascular health; contributes to healthy cognitive function and mood; and can aid in preventing certain cancers. It's just so amazing!

In theory, we should get enough vitamin D just living our lives. Our bodies produce it naturally when our skin is exposed to sunlight (hence its nickname), and it can also be found in a few foods such as fatty fish like salmon, tuna, and sardines, egg yolks, and mushrooms (or in fortified foods like dairy milk and orange juice). Unfortunately, because people spend less time outdoors these days—and because of increased use of sunscreen when we do get outside—about 42 percent of Americans are deficient in vitamin D.

Just like their adult counterparts, newborns are also unlikely to get enough vitamin D from diet alone—be it breast milk or formula—and most parents are not comfortable plopping them down in full sun without protection (*right?*). For this reason, the AAP recommends that all babies less than twelve months of age receive 400 IU of supplemental vitamin D every day, starting shortly after birth until they're weaned (for breastfed babies) or until they begin drinking 32 ounces of vitamin D–fortified formula or whole milk (the milk only after twelve months).

Personally, my stance does differ somewhat from the mainstream guidance regarding vitamin D supplementation for infants. I don't think every baby, without exception, should receive vitamin D supplementation. Given that so many people are vitamin D deficient, there's clearly a problem with the way we are living. We have become *so* sun phobic that we're now lacking a critical vitamin we need to thrive. In my opinion, rather than pile on supplements, the most natural and preferable path to getting the optimal amount of vitamin D is lifestyle change, that is, greater sun exposure.

I know that sounds counterintuitive. And being alert to the dangers of skin cancer and using commonsense caution to do your best to prevent it is a good thing. But we should still be getting out more. And I mean a lot more. We weren't designed to spend the vast majority of our time indoors. Before the Industrial Revolution, when factory and office work became commonplace, people spent *much* more time outside. And vitamin D deficiency was not a major issue.

No, babies should not wear sunscreen. There are appropriate ways to expose them to the sun. The safe way to do so is to get short bursts of sunlight in ten- to twenty-minute walks, early in the morning or in the late afternoon. Sit outside in the shade. Try to increase the natural light in your home, keeping shades and blinds open if appropriate. Of course, don't expose your baby to the midday sun or keep him or her outside for extended periods of time without sun protective clothing. I am absolutely not advocating you let your baby get sunburned. And if you live in a very hot and sunny climate, make sure to prioritize keeping your baby cool and hydrated. Essentially, parents, use your judgment to make the call. You know your kid and his or her skin type best, as well as the climate where you live.

Of course, your baby may be born in the dead of a Minnesota winter or at the height of a Phoenix summer, limiting your ability to safely or comfortably spend time outdoors. In that case, supplementing makes sense. When it comes to selecting which vitamin D drops to give your child, if you choose to do so, you want to make sure that you're giving vitamin D_3. FYI: there are two kinds of vitamin D—D_2 and D_3. Whereas D_2 is the type found in foods, D_3 is the type our bodies produce after exposure to sunlight. Research has shown that, when it comes to supplementation, our bodies absorb D_3 better and sustain higher levels of vitamin D overall with its use. Studies have also shown D_3 is better at stimulating and supporting immune function. In addition, choose drops that are third-party tested (to make sure they are safe and accurately labeled) and avoid any that contain additives or sweeteners. The fewer ingredients the better. Though the standard recommendation is 400 IU per day, I find most parents prefer to just get the 1,000 IU drops and give two to three drops a week.

Omega-3s

Omega-3s are essential fatty acids. They are termed "essential" because our body needs them to function well, although we cannot produce them ourselves. Instead, we derive these essential nutrients from our diet. There are three kinds of omega-3s: DHA, EPA—found primarily in fatty fish like salmon and mackerel—and ALA, which we get mostly from nuts and seeds. Those first two are particularly critical; DHA and EPA are crucial for cell growth and health (the cell membrane is made almost entirely of fatty acids), muscle activity, cardiovascular health, and brain development and function.

If you are thinking about supplementing with fish oil, look for DHA and EPA in the ingredients list. Third-party testing is especially important here; you want to make sure the oil is free of heavy metals (like mercury, which can be prevalent in larger fatty fish) and environmental contaminants. As for the dosage, the FDA hasn't set any guidelines regarding daily value percentages for DHA, EPA, or ALA individually. However, the National Institutes of Health has set a recommended intake of omega-3s overall (i.e., the recommended amount of DHA, EPA, and ALAs combined), for every age. For birth through twelve months, that amount is 0.5 g per day.

Probiotics

You know gut health has gone mainstream when #guttok has over half a billion views on TikTok (never mind that "guttok" sounds like something my grandmother might have said to me after I sneezed). Yes, there's an influencer for everything. Although this in and of itself may not be the best indicator of the direction in which we are headed as a civilization, there's no disputing that an expanding awareness of the central role of the gut microbiome in our overall health is a good thing. There are few tenets of natural-minded—and now mainstream—medicine about which I feel more strongly than the effect of diet on our health. Although adults can (and should) make any number of lifestyle changes to improve their gut health, infants under six months are another story.

Though their gut microbiomes will eventually host trillions of microbial cells by adulthood, babies are born with a gut that is almost sterile. Nature takes care of this by exposing infants to tons of beneficial bacteria during vaginal birth, bacteria that then thrive, in the gut, on the nutrients found in breast milk. While I most certainly do not purport to "shame" any of the following, the evidence shows that c-sections, early antibiotics use, and formula feeding all interfere with the development of the microbiome, and have been linked to increased risks for obesity, asthma, allergies, and autoimmune diseases.

Even breastfed infants aren't immune to the issues of an out-of-whack gut microbiome. Recent research has shown that in industrialized countries (hello, fellow North Americans!), breastfed infants lack a robust amount of the bacterium *Bifidobacterium infantis* (*B. infantis*), typically inherited from mom through breast milk. *B. infantis* is the bacterium that breaks down milk sugars (as well as boosts the immune system). Why does this matter? Well, because no other bacteria besides *B. infantis* are as efficient at digesting milk sugars. Researchers worry that in its absence, the benefits that breast milk confers may become limited, both in terms of developing the microbiome and in overall health—leading to rising cases of issues such as chronic inflammation and immune dysregulation.

Because gut health is now understood to be such a critical piece in the mosaic of overall health, and because it's becoming increasingly clear that establishing a healthy gut happens from our earliest moments, scientists, researchers, and doctors have become especially interested in the possibility of using probiotics to help support and improve it. What are probiotics? They're live microorganisms—bacteria, mostly—that, in theory, alter our gut microbiome for the better and thus benefit our health when we consume them. While there have been promising studies on using probiotics in general, we have a long way to go with the research; there are just so many types of bacteria that understanding which may yield the greatest benefits is a complex task. And the existing evidence is mixed. What is clear from extensive studies, however, is that probiotics are generally considered safe to use. For healthy adults and children, the risks of probiotic use are extremely minimal.

Yet, because solid evidence on the benefits of taking probiotics does not yet exist, I don't recommend routine supplementation of probiotics for infants. That said, there is really good evidence that probiotics may be helpful for specific situations, so I do recommend stashing some in your home wellness kit.

Gripe Water

Back in the nineteenth century, when gripe water first came into wide use, its two main ingredients were alcohol and sugar. I mean, no wonder those old-timey colicky babies quit griping after a nip of this stuff. Alcohol and sugar—especially combined—tend to make most humans less cranky temporarily. Emphasis on temporarily . . . overdoing the combination almost always leads to a world of hurt. Today's gripe water (minus the booze) is still marketed as a panacea for colic, as well as gas, teething, hiccups, and other general baby complaints—though it warrants repeating: *always read the label* of any product you intend to feed your child before giving it to him or her.

Modern gripe water formulations vary from brand to brand, Most often, they consist of a combination of herbs—typically fennel, dill, and ginger—that are thought to ease digestion. If you do choose to try gripe water on your colicky baby, keep in mind that it is effectively an herbal supplement and therefore, like all herbal supplements, is unregulated by the FDA. This means the ingredients in gripe water, the processes used to make it, and a company's claims about its efficacy have zero oversight from any kind of official agency. Accordingly, you will want to look for a highly reputable brand and avoid formulations that contain lots of sugar or other preservatives. In the end, I believe the potential benefits generally outweigh the potential risks—particularly if, in the alternative, you are considering medication, which likely carries with it greater risks. In my opinion, gripe water is an excellent first line option for *mild* symptoms.

SECTION III

From Baby to Toddler

The transition from babyhood to toddlerhood is a monumental shift, not just for your little one but for you as a parent. This phase heralds newfound independence, language skills, and a burgeoning personality. It is also accompanied by its own set of challenges, like tantrums and boundary-testing. During this transformative period, one of the most valuable lessons is learning to parent at your child's unique pace. Trust in his or her individual development and resist the urge to compare your child's milestones with those of other children. By tuning into your child's specific needs and timing, you'll navigate this exciting stage more harmoniously.

Feeding Your Child

Remember that "Mission: Keep Them Alive" you embarked on when you took your bundle of joy home? Turns out, the primary objective (aside from showering your children with love and ensuring a safe environment) is to keep their tiny tummies full. Sounds straightforward, right? Not so fast. Navigating the world of infant nutrition—be it breastfeeding, formula feeding, or transitioning to solids—can feel like walking through a minefield. Fear not! In this enlightening section, we'll delve into the science and the soul of feeding your baby. We'll explore evidence-based practices while emphasizing the importance of making decisions that fit your family's unique needs and sustain parents' mental well-being.

BREAST MILK

In a certain way, feeding a newborn is pretty simple. After all, there are only two options: breast milk or formula. That I am pro-breastfeeding likely comes as no surprise. At this point, it is not merely a "natural-minded" pediatrician point of view—you will be hard-pressed to find any doctor who does not encourage it. Simply put, I believe that if you can and are willing to breastfeed, you should. Admittedly, "can" is a complicated word. For a myriad of reasons, such as milk supply, family dynamics, medical history, mental health, lack of leave from work, inadequate support, or difficult working conditions, among others, many women *cannot* breastfeed. For people who can't or choose not to breastfeed, formula is a huge achievement of modern science—one that allows babies to thrive when breastfeeding isn't an option. The formula shortage that dominated the news in mid-2022 was a stark reminder of just how important formula has become. I emphatically state this because I'm here to support parents, not alienate them. There is no solid, substantial evidence of stark long-term disparities between babies who were breastfed and babies who were not. Breastfeeding is not a fast pass to Ivy League admission.

Breastfeeding does have undeniable advantages and benefits to baby in the short term. Breast milk contains a wealth of ingredients that formula can't mimic—in particular, protective antibodies. The presence of maternal antibodies in breast milk is the biggest difference between breast milk and formula that we know of. Antibodies are a type of protein produced by our immune systems when they encounter antigens—harmful foreign substances like bacteria and viruses. Antibodies fight off and attack antigens. Infants are born with immature immune systems, meaning they don't really have the ability to fight off infection super successfully on their own—their bodies are just starting to produce antibodies. During pregnancy, a mother passes IgG antibodies to her baby through the placenta, but its protective effect begins to wane immediately after delivery. After birth, a mother passes IgA, IgM, and IgG antibodies to her baby through breast milk—especially colostrum. As a baby consumes breast milk, it coats his or her mucous membranes and GI system. IgA antibodies bind to bacteria and viruses on those surfaces, preventing them from entering the bloodstream and causing illness. Formula does not contain antibodies. That's all there is to it. It's just a fact, not a judgment.

Now, maybe you've heard that breast milk is "magical" and "adapts" to create new antibodies in response to a baby's illness. Breast milk is amazing, but it is not "magical"; it's biological. And that's amazing enough! Different environments will contain different antigens at any given time. Since moms and their babies usually occupy the same environment, especially in the newborn period, and they are rarely separated, it's no surprise, whatever antigen a newborn encounters, his or her mom is likely to encounter it too. In this way, the antibodies a baby receives from his or her mother's breast milk are specific and adapted to the bacteria and viruses that baby is likely to encounter. Pretty damn cool.

So, my main takeaway for you—besides that you should try to breastfeed if you can—is *when it comes to breastfeeding, whatever you can do, do.* Every little bit counts. Every drop of colostrum and breast milk gets precious antibodies to your newborn baby, building his or her immunity to and protecting baby from respiratory, gastrointestinal, and other serious illnesses, particularly during those first two months when baby's immune system is still immature and baby is the most vulnerable. You could breastfeed for a week, you could breastfeed for six months—the official recommendation of the AAP (specifically, exclusive breastfeeding)—

you could breastfeed for two years—your baby will receive a variety of immediate benefits from breast milk throughout.

Many of the longer-term benefits of breastfeeding you will see touted as facts—such as a lower incidence of childhood obesity—are not, in fact, proven to be causal. The studies these results are taken from typically show an *association* between breastfeeding and lesser frequency of chronic disorders or higher frequency of traits such as positive IQ performance (let's not even get into the issues of IQ testing as a valid means of assessing intelligence). Correlation is not causation. These studies do not account for the other behaviors of parents who breastfeed, or any differences in education or economic status. In my experience, this kind of messaging is meant to encourage mothers to breastfeed but, instead, it creates a kind of pressure that can actually backfire and cause guilt and shame. I point this out, in part, to lessen the moral compunction to breastfeed, so that, in turn, you feel more encouraged to do it. Even if you don't exclusively breastfeed for six months, I want you to feel empowered to create a foundation of long-term health for your child through the countless other choices you make for them—and for yourself—as a parent.

The fact is, in the United States, over 80 percent of new mothers try breastfeeding and over 60 percent start off exclusively breastfeeding. But by age six months, the percentage of babies receiving any amount of breast milk drops to about half while the percentage being exclusively breastfed falls to just under a quarter. It seems pretty clear that the message that breastfeeding is good for mom and baby is out there and is being heard—*and* that breastfeeding falls off significantly fairly quickly. Breastfeeding can be difficult, and, as I mentioned earlier, there isn't a lot of social support for breastfeeding. As a pediatrician, I don't think moms need more guilt or shame—it's clear that if we want to encourage parents to breastfeed, what they do need is better lactation support, better work leave, greater job security and protections, and better legislation. Those are the things that would truly lead to more breastfeeding, while simultaneously conferring greater benefits and outcomes for all moms and babies.

For parents who do plan to feed their babies breast milk, there are two options: breastfeeding or bottle-feeding pumped milk, done either exclusively or in combination.

BREASTFEEDING

There are about a zillion guides—books, websites, online courses, social accounts, and so on—designed to teach you how to breastfeed and how to solve issues you may encounter while breastfeeding (check out Recommended Resources on page 249 for some of my favorites). I'm not here to address the "how to," though. A wealth of amazing resources on the subject already exists. As always, my number one goal is to help you stress less and do what's right for you, your child, and your family. When it comes to breastfeeding, that means helping to mentally prepare you for it. In my experience, parents are often surprised by—in other words, unprepared for—the challenges breastfeeding can present.

Breastfeeding seems like it should be intuitive, but that isn't necessarily true in all cases. Breastfeeding is a relationship between two people, one of whom is brand new to life and not in full control of even the most rudimentary of his or her basic bodily functions. So, it can take a while to get the hang of things. Now, you might be thinking, "People have been breastfeeding since we first appeared on the African savannas. Parents just want to unnecessarily complicate things these days."

Here's the thing, though: before the rise of industrialization, when people in the West generally lived in or closer to multigenerational family settings, breastfeeding was just as potentially challenging as it is today. But women were surrounded by other women with the requisite experience to guide them through those arduous moments. Their grandmothers, mothers, sisters, in-laws, friends, and community midwives were close at hand to help. Today, most of us in the West no longer have that kind of community around us—and even if we did, many of our parents and grandparents did not breastfeed. It was the norm for many of our parents *not* to do so (my family included).

My best advice to you is, before your baby arrives—take a breastfeeding class. Classes are available at most hospitals that have a labor and delivery department and at birth centers (see Recommended Resources). Both parents should take the class. Have the name of a good lactation consultant on hand. About that . . .

Breastfeeding is both a physical *and* emotional commitment. Whether it comes "easy" or not, it's a lot of work. I say that not to scare anyone off, but to celebrate the labor involved. I also say this because when it doesn't come easily, the challenges can prove emotionally and psychologically taxing. Without the proper support, staying the breastfeeding course may be difficult. Some of the issues you may encounter while getting started on your breastfeeding journey include:

- latching difficulties, including diagnosis of a tongue- or lip-tie;
- milk supply concerns (either too little or too much);
- pain while feeding, including sore or cracked nipples and mastitis; and
- fussiness during feeding or refusing the breast.

One of the single best sources of support, education, encouragement, and help understanding and resolving all of the above is a lactation consultant. Those first few weeks are the most important when it comes to establishing breastfeeding. Working with a lactation consultant can help ensure that you enjoy (although my wife would undoubtedly scoff at my choice of verbiage here) a long and successful breastfeeding relationship with your child.

NAVIGATING THE COMPLEX WORLD OF TONGUE- AND LIP-TIES

If your baby does have difficulty latching, or you regularly experience pain while breastfeeding, your lactation consultant or medical provider might recommend your baby be evaluated for a tongue- or lip-tie. A tongue-tie is the colloquial term for ankyloglossia, a condition in which the strip of tissue that connects the underside of the tongue to the floor of the mouth (the tongue frenulum) is too short or tight, restricting the tongue's movement. A lip-tie is when the tissue connecting the upper lip to the gums (the lip frenulum) is too short and tight, causing restricted movement.

In recent years, more and more parents in my practice have been asking me about tongue- and lip-ties. And in my civilian life as a dad, it seemed like more and more of my friends had babies who'd been diagnosed with a tie and undergone a frenotomy—a surgical procedure in which the frenulum is clipped using a laser or surgical scissors, releasing the tie and allowing for greater mobility. Not wanting to rely just on anecdotal evidence, I checked out the data. It wasn't my imagination: a 2017 study demonstrated a fourfold increase in the number of newborns diagnosed with ankyloglossia and a fivefold increase in the number of frenotomies performed in the United States between 2003 and 2012.

Increasingly, many doctors—myself among them—feel that this increase is less about better diagnosis and more about increased awareness among parents, driven both by social media and a greater emphasis on breastfeeding, coupled with the relative ease of the procedure. As with overmedication, practitioners who may want to deliver the quick fix that some worried parents are looking for can be overzealous in recommending frenotomies, leading to unnecessary intervention. While the potential complications a tie can cause when it comes to feeding and speech development are cause for concern, the question of when the attachment is *actually* an issue is often open for debate. An oral surgeon, a speech therapist, and an ENT may all have a different opinion about the clinical significance of a tie and whether it needs treatment. Let's keep in mind that everyone's tongue and upper lip are *supposed* to be attached to their mouth and gums, respectively. When it comes to lip-ties in particular, the frenulum will change and move as your baby grows and their teeth come in.

Given all this, if you suspect a tie or a practitioner suggests your child may have one, it's crucial to get a comprehensive evaluation from a qualified health-care provider who adopts an integrative and holistic approach and who is not "clip happy." A diagnosis often involves a multidisciplinary team of pediatricians, oral specialists, and lactation consultants who assess not just the physical tether, but also the functional impact it has on your child's life. Just because a procedure can be done, doesn't mean it should be done. I find parents are often, understandably, looking for a fix to their feeding challenges. In the process, they forget that feeding can be hard in the first few weeks and that babies may simply need some time to get the whole feeding thing down.

Additionally, parents often feel pushed into making quick decisions, swayed by frightening scenarios of the feeding difficulties, speech delays, or even craniofacial issues that could befall their child. These concerns are valid. Addressing the serious issues tongue- and lip-ties can cause—especially when basic functions like feeding or speaking are impaired—is important. Yet, no matter how tempting desperate parents may find a quick fix, I strongly caution against rushing into any surgical procedures without first considering the issue from an integrative perspective—one that considers the unique needs and circumstances of each child. Viewing the issue through this lens may obviate an otherwise avoidable surgery while ensuring that those who genuinely require intervention receive appropriate and timely care.

PUMPING

A couple of years ago, at her child's three-month well visit, I asked a mom, Anjali, how breastfeeding was going. "Well, we finally have the hang of breastfeeding," she responded brightly, "but pumping is so much work." Her face sunk. Wanting to better understand the context, I asked her to describe the difficulties she was experiencing with pumping. I reviewed the baby's chart again. She was gaining weight appropriately, and Anjali hadn't previously mentioned issues with milk supply. I also knew their family had decided Anjali would stay home with the baby for the next two years. "To build a stash," Anjali answered. "You know, just in case. I am not having trouble feeding. I just want to make sure we have extra." Anjali had developed the impression that if you breastfeed, you should always have a stash of frozen breast milk on hand. She described seeing her friends' freezers with orderly trays of dated pouches. But Anjali wasn't going back to work outside the home, or otherwise planning on being separated from her baby regularly or at length. I explained that there was no need for her to be pumping so much, if at all.

Peace of mind is great—but Anjali's determination to "build a stash" was creating anything but peace. Instead, she felt burned out and reduced to being a "milk maker" (her words). Eventually, Anjali wasn't even able to use up all the milk she had stashed, ultimately donating what she could. She tossed most of the expiring stash she had worked so diligently to produce and believed she would need. She threw away hours of time spent arduously pumping when she could have spent that time doing anything else instead. And Anjali was just the first of what would become a flow of new parents in my practice who seemed to think routine pumping was just a normal extension of breastfeeding—something they *had* to do.

So, do you have to pump? Do you really need a freezer stash? Pumping definitely has many benefits in specific circumstances. The thing about pumping, though, is that it is enormously time consuming and, from what I'm told, can be uncomfortable. When you have a newborn, there is barely time between feedings to pump and properly cleaning all the parts of a pump is a laborious chore. If breastfeeding is going well, you don't have issues with supply, and you don't plan on being separated from your baby for more than a couple of hours, then no, you don't need to pump. You don't need a freezer stash, or at the least, you don't need an enormous freezer stash. Sure, have a few feedings worth on hand, just in case.

Of course, for a number of moms, the option to pump is a huge boon, and for many, a necessity. If you are going back to work outside the home and want to continue to feed your baby breast milk, you're going to have to pump. If you plan on traveling for work, spending a night out, or taking a vacation without baby (even just a weekend away), you're going to need to pump at some point. If you can't breastfeed, but you can produce breast milk and want to feed it to your baby, you'll need to pump. If you have a low milk supply, pumping may help. If you know ahead of time that any of these scenarios apply to you, invest in a pump before baby arrives. Dedicate some time to figuring out what type of pump makes sense for you. If you're a first-time parent, and your health insurance covers the cost of a pump, there's no harm in having one on hand. The most efficient are electric double pumps, and there are even cordless breast pumps available now. (One mom in my practice told me she pumps while stuck in LA traffic . . . I'm not sure about how safe this is, but wow, did I admire her efficient use of freeway time.) That said, there are many different types of pumps for expressing milk, including manual pumps, which may work better for you if you only plan to pump occasionally.

When to start pumping depends almost entirely on your particular situation. If you know when your maternity leave ends, you can think about starting to pump and building an appropriate stash a few weeks beforehand, so you give yourself time to get the hang of it. Remember though, you only need enough for those first few days or a week, with maybe a bit extra for unforeseen circumstances (like your boss thinking it's perfectly okay to hand you a new project as you're walking out the door at 5:00 p.m.). Ideally, you'll be pumping at work when your baby would normally be feeding, so you'll have his or her replacement feeds ready to go for the next day.

In general, by four to six weeks, breastfeeding should be well established and baby won't necessarily be eating every one and a half to three hours. This means you will most likely have a little extra time between feedings to pump. If you're separated from your baby for medical reasons and/or you need to encourage your milk supply, you may need to start pumping earlier, even soon after birth. Regardless of circumstance, in general the "right" amount of milk to stash is the amount you need to cover your separation from your baby.

PUMPING AND DUMPING

Food and drinks consumed by mom affect her breast milk. It seems pretty obvious, right? You eat or drink something and voilà, it shows up in breast milk. Sort of. When you eat or drink, or ingest something like supplements or medications, your digestive tract breaks down what you've consumed, making the nutrients more available. Your intestines absorb most of the nutrients, which, helped along by specialized cells, then cross the intestinal lining into your bloodstream so that your circulatory system can pass them on to other parts of your body to store or use. I know that sounds a bit medical. (There will be a pop quiz at the end.) Simply put, you should understand that the nutrients you consume can end up in baby's milk. When it comes to breast milk, as the nutrients (or other substances) in your blood flow through the capillaries near your breast tissue, some pass through and enter your milk. This process, called diffusion, is impacted by a huge variety of factors, like how much of a substance survives digestion, the size of the nutrient particles that pass into the blood, and the concentration of them in your bloodstream—just to name a few. Not everything passes into breast milk in equal amounts or at equal rates of speed. Knowing that, let's tackle a popular subject: "pumping and dumping" (PD).

No, "pumping and dumping" is not the latest and greatest dating app. PD is the colloquial term for the act of pumping breast milk and then throwing it away after drinking alcohol. The thinking behind it is that by doing so, you're getting rid of alcohol-"contaminated" breast milk so that you can then safely breastfeed your baby. The problem is, the alcohol level in milk is essentially the same as the alcohol level in your bloodstream (in other words, as long as you have alcohol in your blood, you're going to have alcohol in your milk). The only effective measure for clearing it from your milk is time. PD does not speed up this process. (That said, if you're going to be missing a breastfeeding session, PD will help you maintain your supply and hopefully avoid engorgement.)

Alcohol is typically at its peak level in breast milk for about thirty to sixty minutes after first consuming a drink, but it remains present in your breast milk for about two to three hours. Please note I said "a drink." That's quite literal—those numbers are based on a single drink. The more you drink, the longer alcohol stays in your milk. In general, after two drinks, alcohol will be present in breast milk for about four to five hours; after three drinks, six to eight hours; and so on. But even these numbers are just minimum safety guidelines: the length of time alcohol remains in your blood/breast milk is also heavily influenced by other factors like how much an individual weighs, whether or not they consumed the alcohol on an empty stomach, how fast the alcohol was consumed, and the individual variations from body to body that affect the way each of us metabolizes booze.

Obviously, PD wouldn't be a thing if it weren't for parents' entirely reasonable concerns about how safe—or not—it is for babies to consume alcohol via breast milk. If a baby were to breastfeed while alcohol is present in its mother's milk, the amount of alcohol it would consume would be about 5 to 6 percent of the weight-adjusted maternal dose. This amount would not generally be considered clinically relevant as long as mom had only one drink that day—the definition, per the CDC, of a "moderate" amount of alcohol. In general, "moderate" alcohol consumption (one "standard" drink per day) is considered safe while breastfeeding, especially if you wait to breastfeed for two to three hours after having a drink. But what does "standard" mean? The CDC guidance is based on the Dietary Guidelines for Americans, which are:

12 ounces of 5% ABV beer

5 ounces of 12% ABV wine

1.5 ounces of 40% ABV (80 proof) liquor

This doesn't mean you should go wild or that alcohol is good for your baby, but a drink here or there is probably not going to be problematic. If you do happen to indulge in a glass of wine to handle all of my terrible jokes and puns, you probably don't need to pump and dump. A small amount of alcohol should not be something that majorly stresses you out. Your baby will be just fine if you have one drink with your friends—just ask anyone who grew up in Europe.

When it comes to other recreational substances—THC and CBD products are now legal in an increasing number of locations around the world—there is limited research on their safety during breastfeeding. THC, the psychoactive component in cannabis, can be transferred to your baby through breast milk and may affect the baby's developing brain. And of course, we now know that PD is not a thing. Given these facts, it's advisable to avoid regularly using cannabis, including CBD products that may contain THC, while breastfeeding. And please: always store edibles in a locked container safely out of reach of children and pets. Nobody wants to come home to a baby wearing tie-dye, jamming out to Bob Marley. (I joke, but in all seriousness, with the growing prevalence of CBD and THC consumption, children are increasingly ending up in the hospital with edible toxicity.)

Speaking of things that are no big deal in California, let's talk Botox and fillers. (Ah, from edibles to injectables—just another day in the life of a pediatrician in Los Angeles.) "Hey, doc, is it safe to use Botox while I breastfeed?" and "When can I start getting lip filler again?" are pretty common questions I get asked, even in my natural-minded, integrative practice. Technically, non-surgical cosmetic procedures such as fillers and injectables are considered safe during breastfeeding. But, and allow me to emphasize, there is *very limited* research on this topic. Personally, I feel that if you're breastfeeding, you should avoid getting injectables for as long as possible. Not only will your face and body change a lot over the next year, but also, Botox is a neurotoxin. Common sense dictates that those products won't be considered safe for breastfeeding twenty years from now.

Finally, when it comes to lack of research, there are the issues of vitamins and medications. You should always consult your health-care provider before starting any new medication or supplement, especially when breastfeeding. While many vitamins and medications are considered safe to take while breastfeeding, some medications can enter breast milk and may not be suitable for breastfeeding mothers. When considering whether to take a medication, you must understand that most medications have not been thoroughly studied in breastfeeding or pregnancy. There are some big ethical implications around testing pregnant women, not to mention few who would volunteer for such studies.

In consultation with your doctor, you will need to personally weigh the potentially unknown risks of taking a medication while breastfeeding against the known benefits of that medication to your health. If a medicine or supplement is helpful to you, then the risk may be worth it in your situation. A common example is anxiety and depression medications. While some medicines have a caution warning for breastfeeding, you may truly need your medication, so the clear benefit outweighs the potential risks for you (individualized medicine at its finest). In other instances, the possible risks may not be worth it and you can hold off until you are done breastfeeding. Again, these are not the types of decisions that should be made unilaterally.

LactMed is a great online resource to look up the safety of various drugs (see Recommended Resources).

FORMULA

Breast milk is unequivocally the most nutritious food you can feed your baby. If you're unable or choose not to breastfeed, though, give a huge thanks to science and technology. Before the advent of safe, commercially available formula in the 1950s, breastfeeding issues could be calamitous—

babies starved. Formula is a modern miracle, not something to demonize. Despite the fact that formula makers can't replicate breast milk exactly (amazingly, breast milk is so complex scientists still haven't identified all its components—not to mention the issue of antibodies), babies who rely on formula do just fine. Not only do they survive, they thrive.

Our first goal when it comes to feeding our babies should be ensuring they're getting enough calories and nutrients. That's what "fed is best" means. I will always support breastfeeding as the gold standard of nutrition for newborns. That said, you will never find me proselytizing from high up on my doctor pulpit to convince parents to avoid formula.

Let's talk a little bit about formula. Formula is a lot less complicated than it seems—at least *choosing* a formula, that is. Walk down any formula aisle in the US and you're likely to be overwhelmed by the variety of formulas to choose from. (As I type this, there are more than fifty kinds of formula approved for sale by the FDA on store shelves.) It's no surprise to me that the most common question parents ask me about formula is "Which one should I choose?"

There is no "correct" answer. All formula sold in the United States has to meet the same set of stringent criteria imposed by the FDA. These criteria require formulas to meet very clearly defined nutritional needs and to spell out not only which ingredients formula must and must not contain, but also how it is manufactured. The FDA very tightly monitors and regulates formula—any formula sold in the US will meet a baby's nutritional needs from birth through twelve months. Barring specific medical issues, anything you choose is going to be adequate for your little one in terms of supplying all the nutrients he or she needs to grow and develop. Truly. Oh, and generic and name-brand formulas are virtually identical, except in price. Fun fact: the same four companies manufacture over 90 percent of the baby formula available for sale in the US.

There are three *forms* of infant formula available and three main *types* of formula. The three forms are powdered, concentrated liquid, and ready-made. Powdered formula is measured by the scoop and mixed with a corresponding amount of water—you can make a single bottle or a larger batch. Concentrated liquid is similar to powder in that it must also be measured and mixed with water. Ready-made formula (or ready to use) is just what it sounds like—formula that's been premixed and typically sold in packages of individual four-ounce bottles; its primary use is with newborns. Powder formula is the most widely available, most affordable, and most popular by far, and is what we'll largely be discussing here.

The three types of formula are milk protein–based, soy-based, and protein hydrolysate. Milk-based formulas are the most common and what almost all full-term, healthy babies who formula feed consume. Soy-based formulas are designed for babies with certain medical conditions or whose parents prefer a plant-based alternative. Protein hydrolysate formulas are designed for babies who have milk protein allergies. Unless your pediatrician recommends you feed your baby a soy or protein hydrolysate for medical reasons, you will likely choose from the vast array of milk-based formulas. It should also be noted that some other countries manufacture goat milk formulas. There are a number of non-soy plant-based formulas in the pipeline as well. At this time, these are not approved for US newborns, though I suspect that may change in the next few years.

Given the stringency of FDA requirements and the resultant similarity among formulas, the formula you choose is going to be mostly a matter of preference, boiling down to the price and/or minor differences in ingredients. The basic makeup of most formulas for full-term babies is very similar: most formula is modeled as closely as possible after breast milk and contains a balance of proteins, carbohydrates, fats, vitamins, and minerals. Here's what you should consider:

Protein in formula comes from milk proteins, as it does in breast milk. You might see proteins listed as milk, nonfat milk, whole milk, goat milk, milk protein isolate, whey, or hydrolyzed whey. In soy-based formulas, it will be soy protein. Breast milk contains two types of proteins: whey and casein, in about a 60:40 ratio. Formula also contains whey and casein, but in varying amounts, so you want to look for one that comes close to that 60:40 ratio—this is one of the times Dr. Google can be a good friend.

Whereas in traditional formula for healthy full-term babies, milk proteins are "intact" (in other words, they haven't been broken down), in formulations labeled "gentle," the proteins are "partially hydrolyzed," meaning they have been partially broken down. This makes them closer in size to the proteins in breast milk and, in theory, easier to digest. If your doctor does recommend using a gentle formula, make sure it contains no intact proteins. I know that may seem obvious, but some "gentle" formulas include a mix of intact and partially hydrolyzed proteins, which makes them kind of pointless. If your baby has a diagnosed milk protein allergy, your doctor will likely recommend "hypoallergenic" formula, which contains only fully hydrolyzed, or broken down, proteins.

Carbohydrates are the most abundant substance in breast milk, in the form of the milk sugar lactose. Most formulas replicate this by using lactose from cow's milk. You want to look for formulas that list lactose as the only sugar/carbohydrate. Many baby formulas include other, less expensive carbohydrates in addition to lactose, to meet the FDA's carb requirement. Some include added sugar as a sweetener, to make the formula more palatable. But formula is palatable as is—babies' palates haven't developed yet. If they're hungry, they will eat. Additional sugar is not good for babies (or anyone!), not to mention you're training their palate to prefer sweet food and bias toward high sugar foods as they grow. Other carbohydrates/sugars you might see listed include corn syrup solids, glucose, sucrose, and maltodextrin.

Micronutrients (as opposed to macronutrients, or "macros") in breast milk are directly related to a mother's diet and can vary from feeding to feeding. With formula, there are twenty-nine vitamins and minerals the FDA requires all formula to have, from vitamin A to zinc. Some formulas may contain "extras" that are meant to benefit baby, like DHA or pre- and probiotics—both of which, as we discussed in "A Wellness 'Medicine' Chest for Newborns," are generally considered safe for babies but have mixed evidence when it comes to their benefits. In general, the more "extras" a formula has, the more expensive it is, so I would consider these "nice to haves" rather than necessities.

Stabilizers and emulsifiers like soy lecithin prevent the oil and water in formula from separating once prepared. They're common in all formulas, though organic formulas or European-style formulas may contain sunflower lecithin instead. If you can avoid soy, I always recommend doing so, as nearly all soy produced today is genetically modified. Carrageenan, a seaweed-derived emulsifier, is natural, but remember, natural doesn't always mean good for you. Carrageenan is found in both organic and non-organic baby formulas in the US despite being outlawed for use in infant formula in the European Union. Ready-made varieties of formula tend to have the highest levels of carrageenan.

Organic formula is, like all other formula produced in the US, tightly regulated by the FDA and must meet the same standards as non-organic formula. The big difference is that, in addition to meeting FDA standards, it is certified organic by the USDA. For the USDA to certify formula organic, 95 percent of its listed ingredients must be organic. This means milk-based formulas must use organic milk, which comes from cows that consume pesticide-free feed, are not given antibiotics or growth hormones, and have access to pastures. If you can afford organic formula, I would lean toward using it, especially if this is the only food your child is going to be eating for the first six months of his or her life. Though your baby's exposure to pesticides and antibiotics in non-organic formula may only be in trace amounts, if your circumstances permit you to avoid them entirely, there is no reason not to.

There is no perfect baby formula, but with a little internet searching, you *can* find an FDA-approved baby formula produced in the United States that meets almost all, if not all, of the above criteria. I'm not going to get into brands and products here, because those are ever changing. I can tell you that as I type this, I can confirm that there are several great options on the market, made right here in America. You just have to understand what to look for, read labels, and do a little legwork if necessary (and don't randomly Google "baby formula toxins" and take the word of a blog that, on further inspection, is owned by an organic baby formula company or is published by a third-party European formula reseller). Remember, sources will show you whatever they want to sell to you.

American vs. European Formula

Many of the natural-minded parents I work with are reluctant to use formula even when it's a matter of their baby's health and safety. Once these parents accept that formula is going to be a part of their lives, almost all of them immediately jump to this idea that they'll salvage a less-than-ideal situation by using—trumpets, please—European formula (can't you just see the canister now, bathed in golden sunbeams of wholesomeness?). An increasing number of parents who are far from crunchy are starting to ask me about it as well.

I get it, I do. Our industrialized, hyper profit-driven agriculture and food systems here leave a lot to be desired when it comes to our health (let alone the health of our planet). And the European Food Safety Authority (EFSA) does prohibit or restrict a lot of food additives and preservatives (many linked to cancer) and possible allergens that are still used in the US. The EFSA just has a more proactive—some might say stringent—approach to food safety. They require new ingredients to be tested and proven safe before being added to or sold as foods, whereas in the US food companies are able to introduce additives to foods without much oversight if those additives are deemed "generally regarded as safe," or "GRAS." It's not until they're proven *unsafe* that they're pulled from market (and let's not get into what determines or who decides if an ingredient is, indeed, unsafe). There are good reasons for the lack of trust a lot of people feel.

But infant formula in the US is one of the most strictly regulated and closely monitored food products that exists in this country, as well as being heavily studied and subject to ongoing research. It even has its own law governing its production: the Infant Formula Act of 1980. When it comes down to it, US formula and European formula are not *as* different as some would have you believe. They do have some key differences overall, though—let's get into them.

The first thing you should understand is that, overall, US formula and European formula have the same nutritional profile: they require similar calories per serving and similar percentages of carbohydrates, fats, and proteins and similar vitamins and minerals as part of their composition. Most European Union (EU) formulas meet the nutritional standards of the FDA—obviously, European babies (and a growing number of Americans) thrive on them. The biggest difference lies in how the EU requires formula makers to meet the requirements for carbohydrates. Like the US, the EU also requires formula to be comprised of 40 percent carbohydrates, in order to best match breast milk. But in the EU, 30 percent of *those* carbohydrates must come from lactose. This is not the case in the US (though you can find formulas in the US with lactose as the only carbohydrate). The EU does not allow the addition of certain carbohydrates/sugars, such as corn syrup solids, to regular infant formula, though it does allow others, like maltodextrin, so it is just as important to read the labels of EU-produced formula.

When it comes to vitamins and minerals, the FDA and the EFSA agree on the basics, but are far apart on two major points. The first disagreement is how much DHA and iron formula should have. The EU requires formula to contain a certain amount of DHA, whereas the US does not require it to have any, though many US formulas now include DHA as a selling point. Personally, I don't think the inclusion of DHA makes EU formula "better." It certainly doesn't make it "cleaner" or "greener." As we discussed in "A Wellness 'Medicine' Chest for Newborns," the current evidence of the benefits of omega-3 supplementation for infants is mixed, and you can always choose to supplement if your formula does not contain DHA. The US also requires much higher levels of iron in infant formula than the EU does. The goal is to prevent iron deficiency anemia, which can have serious developmental consequences.

The second disagreement pertains to genetically modified organisms (GMOs). The EU prohibits the use of GMO ingredients in its formulas, along with carrageenan and certain synthetic preservatives and additives like lutein, beta-carotene, taurine, nucleotides, and L-carnitine, that the US does not. These additives are meant to mimic some of the bioactive components of breast milk, but research does not fully support their benefits in formula. There are formulas available in the US that do not include these additives (or GMO products)—again, this is an instance where you need to read your labels. EU formula does include emulsifiers and stabilizers, but generally you will see the use of something like sunflower lecithin rather than soy lecithin because of the prohibition on inclusion of GMO products. I mention this because in your internet deep dive, you may read that EU formula doesn't contain the "nasty" ingredients that are in US formulas, like stabilizers and emulsifiers. This is my reminder to you that the internet often lacks nuance, let alone accuracy.

In my mind, one of the greatest advantages EU formula offers parents in Europe is choice. There are many more milk-based options available there, including goat milk– and whole milk–based formulas, formulas that meet pasture-raised requirements (not just organic requirements), and gentle formulas that still rely on lactose as their sole carbohydrate (which is currently not the case in the US). There are also more choices with regard to the type of oil used. In the US *and* EU, most formulas use palm oil. More recently, a number of newer formulas in the EU are using alternative oils, such as coconut, sunflower, and safflower. Which oil is "best" remains subject to debate. The bottom line is that the EU offers more choices to meet your personal preference. EU parents don't need to read their formula labels quite as closely, because they can rest easier knowing that certain ingredients are simply not allowed.

So, why can't I wholeheartedly recommend and support the use of third-party imported EU formula here? Well, it's largely because of that "third party" piece. EU formula is not regulated by the FDA, so technically it is not legal to sell in the US. This means that in order to purchase it, American parents must buy it from third-party resellers—Holle and HiPP can't just ship it directly to your local Target. These resellers have no oversight—we have no way of knowing how the formula was stored or handled on its way to us, which are both quality and safety issues. Consequently, American parents have a much tougher time knowing if a European manufacturer has issued a recall—which does happen.

The other big downside to European formula for Americans, is that the instructions regarding its preparation and storage are not always in English (and their scoop size and thus the water ratio are not the same as US formulas). This leaves room for error, with the potential of either feeding your baby formula that is too diluted or too concentrated. Finally, it is just a lot more expensive. Given its cost, it is simply not a good option for many families.

Look, we all know the allure of all things European: gooey cheese! Great public transportation! Subsidized health care! Cobbled streets! But, I promise, European formula is not the only acceptable formula for your bébé. Armed with your knowledge of what formula is made of and why, along with what you should look for and avoid, you *can* find a US formula to meet your needs that is organic, free of GMOs, and lactose based. It simply takes a little extra effort—which is seemingly well worth it. After all, you're reading this book because you're a discerning parent who cares about your child's health.

Making Your Own Formula

I would be remiss if I did not touch upon the supremely crunchy topic of making your own formula. To my surprise, this topic is being raised more frequently by the parents in my practice. If you're wondering about this as a possibility, wonder no longer, dear reader: do *not* make your own formula.

I don't blame you for wishing to become a formula mixologist. I do not recommend it, though. The parents I know who have attempted to make formula (or were planning on doing so before I counseled them otherwise) truly have the best intentions. They typically ask, "How can something artificial that is mass produced in a factory be better than something I could make at home with the freshest, cleanest ingredients?" But making your own formula can be extremely dangerous for your child.

The problem lies in the very simple fact that breast milk—and its closest imitator, formula—is incredibly complex nutritionally. It's so complex that even after decades and decades of research, scientists are still studying it, hoping to learn more about its properties and the ways they support, adapt to, and influence human development. While formula can't match that complexity, it is carefully designed to match the nutritional profile of breast milk—to provide not only calories, but the *right types* of calories, and the right amounts of specific vitamins, minerals, and other bioactive compounds.

Homemade formula is almost guaranteed to be nutrient deficient in some way. The "recipes" of commercially available formulas are based on the joint knowledge and research of many types of scientists, from experts in neonatology to nutrition to brain development . . . you get the picture. It would be near impossible for one person to be in full possession of all the knowledge that goes into making sure formula has all the necessary ingredients for an infant to thrive. A good example would be fat. Sounds simple, right? Wrong. The fat content in formula isn't merely intended to meet a percentage. The fat in breast milk contains a range of particular fatty acids, including, among others, palmitic and oleic acids. There is no single vegetable oil that matches the fatty acid profile of breast milk, so formula manufacturers use a *combination* of different oils to match it as closely as possible. Even with a medical education, I am ill equipped to concoct a fat blend in my home kitchen that correctly combines the right medium- and long-chain saturated and unsaturated fatty acids.

The nutrient deficiencies that can occur with use of homemade formula are not to be taken lightly. Formula may likely be the *only* source of nutrition a young baby receives for many consecutive months. A "small mistake" can have devastating consequences. When I was a resident physician at Children's Hospital Los Angeles, a six-month-old baby came in with a terrible rash over large areas of his body, with blisters around his mouth and diaper area. This sweet baby looked severely sunburned and was in apparent distress. His parents were confounded. As far as they knew, their child hadn't encountered or consumed any known allergens, and they had definitely been diligent about shielding him from sun exposure. It turned out the baby was suffering from a serious zinc deficiency. His well-meaning parents wanted to breastfeed, but were unable to do so. In their effort to avoid commercial formula, they concocted their own formula from recipes on the internet. This mix did not deliver the requisite amount of zinc human infants need to function. In an effort to protect their child from what they perceived to be the "dangers" of commercial formula, these clearly well-intentioned parents may have inadvertently caused irreparable harm to their child. Luckily we were able to provide the needed vitamins and the baby quickly recovered. But if the family had not come to the hospital when they did or we did not figure out the underlying cause of the rash, the ending may not have been a happy one.

A zinc deficiency isn't "just" a matter of a rash (that's the clinical manifestation of it). Zinc is a mineral that has a tremendous part in the healthy functioning of the human body. It plays a role in cell growth, brain structure development (and thus brain function), GI tract development, protein metabolism, immune function, reproduction, and wound repair, to name a few. The tricky thing about zinc is that even though it exists in abundance in our bodies, we can't really store it in significant amounts—so we need to continuously re-up our supply, either through supplementation or by eating zinc-rich foods. For a baby, that means breast milk or formula. Prolonged zinc deficiency can lead to a lot of horrible outcomes including permanently stunted growth and development, liver disease, endocrine disorders, and cognitive impairment.

And that's just one of the twenty-nine vitamins and minerals the FDA requires, in specific amounts, be present in infant formula. This is one of those moments when even the skeptics among us must humbly acknowledge that infant formula is an amazing scientific achievement. Science has come a long way to create a substance that can keep babies alive and nourish them well—many millions of babies in the US have been formula fed and are alive and healthy. Yes, we can always make it better. Maybe in five hundred or even fifty years future generations will consider today's formula a quaint relic of old-timey science. Formula may not be "perfect," but that does not mean it is bad. It's fine to be skeptical. Heck, as a rule, I applaud skepticism and always encourage parents to ask questions. Nevertheless, the cold, hard fact is that there is a lot of brain power invested into, well . . . formulating formula. And new formulations, with wider options for organic and European-style formulas, are emerging all the time. The push for cleaner, healthier ingredients works—but pushing for better formula should not be mistaken for rejecting currently available formulas outright.

I must emphasize: feeding your baby homemade formula is taking a huge gamble with his or her health and, potentially, life—even if you scooped a generous helping of best intentions into the recipe. This is one situation in which trying to be all "natural" all the time can have dire repercussions and simply isn't worth it in my opinion.

Safe Formula Preparation and Storage

As should be evident to you by now in any discussion regarding infant formula, safety is the biggest concern. This rings all the more true when it comes to the preparation and storage of formula. There are two biggies right out of the gate that might make you say "duh!":

1. Do not use expired formula.
2. Wash your hands before you prep it.

Obvious, right? Yet, when it comes to the former, you would be surprised how many people forget to check the expiration date before using formula. Yes, you just bought the can yesterday at the local big-box store. Although unlikely, it could still be expired. Always check the expiration date. Using expired formula could subject your child to possible illness. The USDA requires that all infant formula be marked with a "Use By" date, and that "consumption by this date ensures the formula contains not less than the quantity of each nutrient as described on the label." In other words, expired formula may no longer meet your child's nutritional needs.

When it comes to preparing formula, the most frequently asked question I hear is "What kind of water should I use?" In the US, most parents have access to at least one of these two water sources:

- Bottled water: I am not a fan of using plastic bottled water to mix formula. (And don't get me started on "Nursery Water." You don't need it. This is just another unnecessary gimmick intended to separate parents from their money.) Most bottled water comes in plastic bottles and is just tap water masked as something fancier. A 2018 study that tested many of the most popular bottled water brands in the US and abroad found that 93 percent of them contained microplastics. While microplastics are sadly becoming more and more prevalent in our environment, the study found that there was about twice as much plastic in bottled water as there was in tap water. Plastics contain endocrine-disrupting chemicals (EDCs) that are less than ideal for human health. EDCs are linked to cancer, diabetes, reproductive disorders, and neurological impairments of developing fetuses and children, among other negative outcomes. Bottled water also leads to high amounts of plastic waste, leading to more microplastic contamination in our environment. In my opinion, plastic bottled water is best reserved for instances where you know your drinking water source is unsafe. If you are able to get water bottled in glass, especially spring water, that is often the source of water with the lowest amount of chemicals. Of course, it is not always accessible or financially viable.

- Tap water: We are so lucky that the majority of us have access to clean, safe tap water. If you are unsure about your local water quality, you can call your county health department or state environmental agency for more information. In general, good old tap water is fine to use for mixing baby formula. Having a household or personal water filtration system is an added benefit, and any reputable filter will remove some percentage of the unwanted chemicals that remain in tap water. For babies under two months (or babies who are immune compromised), you should boil tap water first, allow it to cool for five minutes but no more than thirty, and then use it to mix formula—this is to ensure that the water is hot enough to kill any cronobacter (a bacteria that can sometimes be found in powdered formula) in the powder. Once you mix a bottle using boiled-then-cooled water, shake a few droplets on your inner wrist to test that it's not too hot for your baby. If it's hotter than body temp, run the bottle under cool water.

After feeding your baby a bottle of prepared formula, throw away whatever is left after an hour. Never put a partially used bottle back in the fridge to finish later. A partially used bottle is a breeding ground for bacteria.

SOLID FOODS

Introducing solids to your baby is a significant milestone for all parents (especially if you're a foodie like me). Obviously we all need to eat to survive, but food is about so much more than survival or even health. Through food we share and preserve our family traditions and cultures; we explore other cultures; we celebrate, create memories, bond, and welcome guests—strangers and friends alike. Through food, we draw close to nature; through food, we experience beauty and pleasure. I would venture to guess that, if I asked any one of you right now, you'd be able to recount your favorite dish from childhood—something a family member prepared or that one thing you always ordered at the "special occasion" restaurant. As a child, mine was my mom's chicken parmesan. As you may have guessed, these days I eat very differently.

When our children begin their journey with solids, we're welcoming them into this essential human experience. I think it's pretty special, something to enjoy—cherish even. And it *really* doesn't have to be complicated.

You've probably heard you should introduce solids at six months—that's when most parents kick things off. There's nothing magical about this number, though. There's no overnight "ready for solids!" switch that gets flipped when the clock rolls over to midnight on day 182.5 of your baby's life. It's just that six months is when most babies typically show the telltale signs that they're ready for solids:

- They can hold their head up well and overall have strong neck and head control.

- They can move food from the front of their tongue to the back of their mouth and their gag reflex is decreasing and moving to the back of their mouth.
- They're interested in food—they watch you intently when you eat, they reach for your food, they open their mouth when food comes their way.
- They can sit *supported by you or a chair* (it's a common misconception that a baby needs to be sitting independently before starting solids—most babies are not sitting on their own at six months, so I'm not sure where this rumor started . . . especially given it predated the all-knowing internet).

If your baby isn't six months yet, but is showing these signs of readiness, it's fine to try solids. I wouldn't start any earlier than four months, though. (If you do want to start on the earlier end, I love mesh or silicone fresh food feeders—they look like pacifiers, but instead of a nipple to suck on, they have a pouch you can fill with soft fruits, like raspberries or bananas, for baby to mouth without the risk of choking, which is awesome . . . cleaning them is a little less awesome.)

Purees vs. Baby-Led Weaning

When it comes to how to introduce solids, there are two basic options: spoon-feeding (purees) or baby-led weaning. There's not much to "explain" when it comes to purees. You mash or blend soft or soft-cooked foods and spoon-feed them to your child. It's an age-old method that has worked for countless generations. If you offer baby a taste of something and he or she pushes it—or lets it fall—out of his or her mouth, that's normal; baby has been on a liquid diet, after all. The texture and thickness of solid food takes some getting used to. You might want to wait another week or so and try again. In any case, start with just a spoonful. The first few times you may mix the food with breast milk or formula. It's totally okay if most of the food ends up *on* your baby (or the floor), rather than *in* your baby. (There's this really great invention called the "bib." Top scientists designed it for this exact purpose.) There's a saying: "Food before one, just for fun." Introducing solids is not really about nutrition; baby should still be getting the vast majority of his or her nutritional needs met through breast milk or formula. It's about teaching baby *how* to eat and building a relationship with food.

Now, if you've had a baby in the last five years and ever dipped a toe in the stormy waters of "parenting" social media, or the infamous "mom groups" of Facebook, then you've probably encountered the term baby-led weaning (BLW), along with the high emotions surrounding it. With BLW, you skip spoon-feeding (and thus purees) entirely and allow baby to self-feed whatever you're eating, as long as it is developmentally appropriate and properly prepared (i.e., sliced safely). The term "weaning" in this context doesn't mean giving up breastfeeding or formula, but rather introducing complementary foods.

The three key principles of BLW are:

- Baby Is in Control: Babies decide what, how much, and how quickly to eat.
- Whole Foods: Instead of purees, babies are given soft foods they can hold and mouth or chew.
- Shared Family Meals: Ideally, babies eat what the family eats (with some modifications for safety and health), when the family eats, promoting a sense of community during mealtimes.

BLW has become increasingly more mainstream over the last few years, promulgated by online content creators who have carved out niches in the baby and toddler spaces. Studies, though limited, have pointed to possible benefits, such as:

- Development of Motor Skills: BLW can promote the development of hand–eye coordination, chewing, and fine motor skills as babies learn to grasp and control the food he or she eats.
- Better Regulation of Hunger Cues: Some research suggests that BLW babies might develop better appetite control and recognition of satiety cues, which could potentially reduce the risk of overweight issues later in life. However, more comprehensive studies are needed to confirm this.
- Familiarization with a Variety of Foods: Early exposure to various textures, flavors, and food groups can help establish broad dietary preferences.

Many parents enjoy doing BLW. It may prove less difficult than making purees, and it's fun to introduce kids to different flavors (and of course, textures) than would otherwise exist in ready-made purees. But BLW can also be a lot of work. There's definitely a learning curve, with a good amount of research needed on how to cut different foods safely for babies at different ages and which foods to avoid entirely. Mealtimes must be very closely supervised to reduce the risk of choking and ensure foods are of appropriate size and texture.

I think it was Shakespeare who said, "To B(LW) or not to B(LW)? That is the question." If you want to attempt BLW, go for it! It can be a great way to spend focused time with your baby, and there is little evidence, based on self-reporting, that it leads to greater frequency of choking than spoon-feeding—one of parents' common fears around it. When it comes to deciding between purees or BLW, families should do what works for them. Online, though, die-hard advocates of BLW can make it seem like if you don't do BLW, your baby is a lost cause, a Philistine-in-the-making who will only ever eat chicken nuggets. BLW is the new "in" choice, but it seems to cause a lot of the new parents I know anxiety, generating a sense of pressure. Don't worry about what others are doing. You know your baby best. Do whatever is right for him or her.

A few months ago, at a well visit for a six-month-old baby, I met with a mom wracked with anxiety about introducing solids to her daughter. She was literally losing sleep worrying about what to do and wanted my advice. The source of her stress? Whether or not to feed her baby purees or, instead, to do BLW.

Ashley, baby Harper's mom, explained to me that she really wanted to do BLW, but had an extreme fear of Harper choking. BLW can involve a lot of gagging, and every time Harper gagged, Ashley panicked. Correction—she would have a full-on panic attack. Not only was this less than ideal for Ashley, it created a lot of stress for her partner and probably for Harper too. As a result, she started feeding Harper mostly purees.

I asked Ashley the reason she wanted to do BLW, and why she felt guilty feeding Harper purees. She began by telling me how she knew BLW was so much "better" for kids and how terrible she felt taking the "easy" route. She described watching adorable babies self-feeding on Instagram and listening to oral-motor experts on podcasts describe the importance of "mouth mapping" (via BLW) for oral development.

In working with Ashley, I shifted her focus to the foundational SEEDS of well-being. Harper's sleep was great—she had just started sleeping through the night without feeding. Considering that the majority of her calories still came from formula and breast milk (as is appropriate at six months), the way she was fed had little impact on her sleep (i.e., she would still be going to sleep on a full tummy).

When it came to exercise—which at six months is really about activity—Harper was getting a lot of tummy time, sitting independently, grabbing objects, actively played in her playpen and was holding her head up. In these ways, she was a good candidate for both BLW and purees.

In regard to Harper's environment, the quality was less optimal. At Harper's age, the most important indicator of a healthy environment for her (when it came to the introduction of solids) was the quality of the interactions at the kitchen table. Despite the adjustable Scandinavian high chair, BPA-free silicone bibs, and stainless-steel toddler utensils, BLW was adding significant stress to mealtimes. Stress is contagious. Ashley's panic attacks were detrimental to her and, consequently, negatively impacted Harper.

Next, Ashley and I discussed diet, or what Harper was eating. This should be the primary concern when introducing solids. Spoon-feeding versus BLW, or engaging in some combination of the two, *will not* determine your child's long-term well-being. The type and quality of food your child eats *will*, as will the habits he or she develops around food. Harper was still primarily breastfed, and would be for the next six months. Whether via spoon feeding or BLW, at this stage, feedings were more about laying the groundwork for long-term health. I urged Ashley to prepare a variety of healthful foods, a rainbow of colors, that would develop Harper's palate. I explained when choosing organic really matters (and when it doesn't).

I also reassured Ashley that feeding Harper purees is far from "taking the easy way." First, there is nothing wrong with doing "less work" when the outcome for your kid is positive either way. You are already doing the most critical work—caring for your child, caring about your child, feeding your child and keeping him or her alive. Parents already experience so much pressure. In particular, moms feel the need to be "perfect." You are not in competition with any other parent.

Ultimately, Ashley and I devised a feeding plan that was manageable and felt good to her, her partner, and Harper. She and her partner made a few purees themselves, whizzing fresh fruits and simple steamed veggies in a blender. They signed up for a fresh puree delivery service that offered a bit more variety and reduced the labor load for the two working moms. She and her partner chose one new food every few weeks that they were excited to introduce to Harper, BLW- style. When I saw them again three months later, Ashley had fed Harper a kale smoothie bowl for breakfast that morning. (Yes, I live in Los Angeles and kale smoothie bowls are a thing.) Harper had tried some mango spears at lunch. Mealtime stress was at a minimum and Ashley stopped worrying about how to feed her baby (and, thankfully, muted the BLW posts in her social media feed).

Here's the thing: BLW is not objectively better than spoon-feeding. It most certainly has a whiff of moral superiority about it, especially among natural-minded parents. Ashley seemed surprised when I told her she did not need to do BLW, especially if it caused her so much grief.

Yes, promoters of BLW point to claims that it reduces the risk of childhood obesity, works to prevent picky eating, and develops a child's social interactions through shared mealtimes. These are big claims, and ones that feel high stakes. But the evidence to support these claims of long-term benefits primarily shows correlation, rather than causation. In other words, any measurable outcomes could be attributed to a zillion other differences in the households that practice it. There is *no* evidence that shows babies who are spoon-fed purees have negative long-term outcomes compared to babies who self-feed. Sure, in BLW, baby chooses when to stop eating. But you can (and should) watch your baby's cues when you spoon-feed too. Moreover, there is no reason you can't do a mix of the two, taking into account your own comfort levels and household resources. You *absolutely* can do both. I have never come across any data that suggests the two methods in combination fail to provide the benefits of either alone.

The introduction of solids should not be such a controversial topic (welcome to the twenty-first century—where seemingly *everything* is a controversial topic, even when it isn't). Every baby is different. There is no singular "right" way to feed your child, particularly when there exist multiple ways to do so safely. For some families, food insecurity *is* the stress. The last thing on this parent's mind is to puree or BLW. We have the luxury of making such decisions for our children, free from any pressure that we are making the wrong decision. There is no wrong decision, so let's reserve our stress for things that actually warrant it.

Personally, I'm a fan of doing both—but your kiddo will do great either way. When it came to Eli, we started with purees and soft foods that were easily mashed. Eli's very first food was actually a small lick of hummus from my favorite restaurant in Los Angeles. From that moment forward, he was well on his way to becoming a baby gourmand.

There is a high likelihood that your parents (and their parents before them) chose rice cereal as your first food. For generations, rice cereal reigned supreme as one of the most popular ways to introduce solids to infants, for obvious reasons. It was economical, convenient, easy to mix with breast milk or formula, and gentle on baby's tummy. In recent years, though, rice cereal has lost some of its luster (okay, a lot of its luster) due to worries around heavy metals and toxins (like arsenic) in rice, along with greater concerns about the negative health impacts of processed foods and GMO products. We did not use rice cereal with Eli, but I'm not strongly opposed to it if you want to start with it. In general, I wouldn't recommend it. I would start with "real" food.

Avocados are a great first food even if you're not a Californian, because you don't have to do any work. With no blending required, avocados meet the criteria for decreased stress. Avocados easily mash or cut into small bites for BLW (though they may be a bit slippery for baby, who's likely still using a palmar grasp at this point). Other simple first foods that are easy to mash, puree, or use with BLW include soft-cooked carrots, soft-cooked peas, or berries like raspberries (blueberries should be completely mashed or blended as their round shape can present a choking hazard).

Whatever you start with, you should introduce new foods one at a time, every two to three days. This way, you can watch for any potential allergic reactions. If you're serving baby a three-ingredient puree of foods they've never had before, you're not going to know which one caused that rash on his or her chin. Once you know that baby has no issue with

DR. GATOR'S FAVORITE FIRST FOODS

Kick-start your little one's journey into the world of solids with Dr. Gator's Favorite First Foods.

Avocado: Rich in heart-healthy fats, buttery flavor, and a creamy texture.

Banana: High in fiber and potassium. Naturally sweet and soft in texture.

Sweet Potato: High in fiber, antioxidants, minerals, and vitamins including A, B_6, C, and manganese. Can be mashed easily once baked or steamed.

specific foods, feel free to combine them. Have fun with it: a carrot and turnip mash, an apple-cranberry puree, pureed chickpeas and zucchini with a little yogurt. Why not?

Do try your best to acquaint your baby with a variety of new foods over time. Encourage your baby—and then your toddler—to "eat the rainbow" by introducing him or her to an array of fruits and vegetables in different colors. Take your child with you to the store or farmers market. Plant a few veggies at home. As your child grows older, ask him or her to pick out foods of different colors. Make it a game. Colorful fruits and veggies are full of vitamins, minerals, flavonoids, antioxidants, and fiber.

To maximize the health benefits from fruits and vegetables, consider feeding your child a colorful variety. Red options like tomatoes and strawberries are rich in antioxidants and vitamin C. Orange and yellow choices such as carrots and mandarins offer a load of vitamin A and beta-carotene. Greens, like spinach and broccoli, are packed with iron, calcium, and folate. Don't overlook blue and purple foods like blueberries and eggplant, which are filled with powerful antioxidants. Lastly, white vegetables like cauliflower, garlic, onions, and mushrooms provide an array of beneficial compounds, including flavonoids, selenium, and vitamin B_6.

FOODS TO AVOID

Honey: As a natural-minded doctor, I'm all about honey. It is a pretty incredible food in many ways—from its ability to soothe and suppress coughs to its wound-healing properties. As a sweetener, it is exponentially better for us than table sugar (though it should still be consumed in moderation). But honey for children under a year old is a huge NO. That includes all cooked, baked, or processed foods that contain honey, like graham crackers. Why? Honey may contain a bacterium called

Clostridium that causes infant botulism. Botulism can cause muscle weakness, trouble swallowing, and trouble breathing and requires hospitalization for infants. (Think about it, that's literally what Botox—an injectable form of botulism—does: it freezes your facial muscles.) Read labels and please avoid giving honey to a baby before he or she is one year old. If your baby does accidentally ingest a little honey, don't freak out. You should tell your doctor and you should monitor the baby for the above symptoms, but developing botulism after eating honey is very rare. I have had many frantic calls from parents after grandpa Karl gave some honey to little Sandra. I have never once seen it turn into botulism.

Sugar: Added sugar has no nutrient value for babies, and an excess of it can lead to a number of chronic health problems. Babies also already have an innate preference for sweetness—remember, breast milk's most abundant nutrient is carbohydrate in the form of lactose, that is, milk sugars—which can be reinforced, to their detriment, by exposure to added sugars. When it comes to solids, you want to help your baby develop an enjoyment of savory foods, as well as naturally sweet foods like fruit. Introducing them to natural tastes without the influence of refined sugar helps set the stage for healthy eating habits. Ideally, it's best to hold off on foods that contain added sugar.

Salt: Infants have immature kidneys and can process only a tiny amount of salt—an amount already found naturally in whole foods and in breast milk. There is no need for you to add salt to their food; in fact, you should generally avoid doing so. As with sugar, we don't want to train our kids' palates to sense food as "flavorful" only if it is salted. Allow them to experience the lovely subtleties of whole foods. Just because something tastes "bland" to you doesn't mean your baby experiences it in the same way.

You wouldn't add salt to breast milk, would you? I do often get asked by parents of older babies—closer to one year—whether it's okay to give a little salt. Typically, this is in the context of giving the baby food from a meal prepared for the parents, as opposed to whipping up a separate, saltless meal for baby. If it makes your life easier, I think a little salt is okay, but I wouldn't make a habit of adding salt to baby's food.

Spices and Seasonings: Although spices and herbs are generally healthy, I suggest introducing them only *after* you've established a good relationship with the base food—think, adding cinnamon to pureed apples after you establish your baby will eat pureed apples, or adding turmeric to lentils after baby has enjoyed lentils several times. At that point, if you do want to try an herb or a spice, add only a pinch and just one herb or spice at a time. It's great to expand your baby's palate with natural and wholesome ingredients like herbs and spices, but again, you want to be mindful of food allergies and sensitivities.

The Dirty Dozen: Every year, the Environmental Working Group (EWG) tests thousands of samples of conventionally grown (i.e., non-organic) fruits and vegetables to see which rank highest and lowest for pesticide residues. The fruit and vegetables that have the most pesticide residue are labeled "The Dirty Dozen." The list can change from year to year, so it's best to look up it yourself annually (though as of this writing, strawberries have topped it at number one for many years). If you can't afford the cost or don't want to spend the extra money on their organically grown counterparts, it's best to avoid the produce on The Dirty Dozen. If that's the case, you can focus on filling those holes in your kiddo's diet with the EWG's "Clean Fifteen," which, you guessed it, is their list of conventionally grown produce that rank *lowest* for pesticide residue. Strong evidence has shown links between pesticide exposure and cancers, as well as other health issues including negative neurologic and reproductive effects.

Water: Okay, I know this one isn't "solid," but it is important to mention that, in general, babies under a year old should not drink water. Breast milk or formula provides all the necessary hydration they need. While small sips of water every now and then might be fine, especially in hot weather, the vast majority of their fluid intake must come from breast milk or formula. It's not that there is something inherently toxic about water—obviously, if you're formula feeding, you are mixing it with water. Water itself is not exactly the issue. Giving a baby too much water can lead to water intoxication, a serious condition in which his or her electrolyte balance becomes disrupted. Filling up on water can also decrease a baby's appetite for breast milk or formula, which could lead to inadequate nutrient intake.

Food Allergies

Most of the parents I work with share one major concern when it comes to starting solid foods, and it's *not* whether to spoon-feed or baby-led wean. It's food allergies. It's completely natural for parents to be cautious about food allergies: they can be dangerous, of course, and really limit certain aspects of our children's lifestyle (and therefore our own). Still, it's important to know that only about one in seventeen kids will be diagnosed with a food allergy, and that two of the most common food allergies among children—milk and eggs—often resolve over childhood. (In the US, the most common food allergens are milk, eggs, peanuts, tree nuts, soy, wheat, shellfish, and sesame; among children specifically, the most common allergen is milk, followed by egg and then peanut.)

The good news is that reams of high-quality recent research suggests that introducing allergenic foods early—before one year of age—rather than avoiding them, may reduce the risk of developing allergies to those foods.

When it comes to introducing allergenic foods, you want to follow the same three-day rule you would with any other food: introduce only one allergenic food at a time and wait three days before introducing another allergenic food. There are a bunch of companies out there that sell specially designed allergenic powders you can add to purees, breast milk, or formula as a way to introduce them to your child's diet. I'm not a huge fan of this method since it means relying on a processed powder. Whenever possible, I think the best choice is to give baby all-natural, whole foods. For some parents, though, the consistent nature of these products can give them a sense of control and lessen anxiety.

Once you introduce an allergenic food to your child, it's important to watch for signs of a food allergy. Food allergy symptoms generally show up within thirty minutes, though it can be as little as two minutes or as long as two hours, and they fall into three basic categories:

Skin: hives, redness, itching, swelling of the mouth or tongue

Respiratory: shortness of breath, hoarse voice/vocalizations, wheezing

Gastrointestinal: vomiting, diarrhea, abdominal pain

Symptoms can appear alone or in combination, and range in severity. If your baby develops a rash, but is otherwise fine, call your doctor. It's helpful to take some photos to document the rash. The doctor may suggest giving your baby an over-the-counter antihistamine. In any case, it's important to make a follow-up appointment with an allergist as soon as possible—your pediatrician should be able to make this referral quickly. Not only is it more likely your little one may have another food allergy, but you do want to confirm that the rash (or other symptom) is, indeed, a food *allergy* and not a food *intolerance*. An allergy provokes an IgM immune response, while an intolerance—though similar in terms of symptoms—does not involve an IgM response.

If your child has trouble breathing, develops hives, passes out, experiences severe stomach pain, or has any other severe symptoms—that is, anaphylaxis—take them to the ER *immediately*.

I know the above scenario is terrifying, but keep in mind that only a very small percentage—0.04–1.8 percent of kids—has ever had a serious anaphylactic reaction to food. For those parents that know someone who has had a serious reaction and live in fear of it happening to their own kids, or just for any parent extremely nervous about introducing allergenic foods (especially peanuts) to his or her child, here's my best piece of advice (it always makes parents smile): Drive to your nearest ER. Find a nearby park or somewhere close to take a stroll. Give your child the food to try. Worst-case scenario, you are right near an ER. The wisdom goes: if you're near the hospital, you won't need it.

Once you know an allergenic food is "safe," the key is to keep introducing it to your child's diet. It's important to eat these foods regularly, because regular exposure to them is important for maintaining tolerance.

Growing and Changing

The early years of life are a period of remarkable growth and change for young children. This stage is a time of physical development, cognitive advancements, and emotional and social maturation. As a parent or caregiver, it's essential to recognize that every child develops at his or her own pace. While it's tempting to compare your child's milestones to those of others, the importance of parenting at your child's pace cannot be overstated.

Well visits to the pediatrician become particularly crucial during this period, serving not only as a preventative health-care measure, but also as a way to track and discuss developmental milestones. These visits offer valuable insights into your child's growth trajectory and individual needs, allowing you to adapt your parenting approach accordingly.

Language development is a significant focus in the first few years, with children's vocabulary and comprehension skills blossoming exponentially. This linguistic growth aids in cognitive development and social interaction, setting the stage for more complex thoughts and relationships. By tuning into these pivotal areas of development, you can create a nurturing environment that supports your child's unique journey toward overall well-being.

WELL VISITS

Early childhood is a critical time for both growth and development, making regular well visits essential for a holistic approach to pediatric care. As a parent, you're not just keeping tabs on your child's physical health during these appointments; you're also laying the foundation for a lifetime of well-being. If adults make it to a yearly physical, they're doing pretty well when it comes to preventive health care. Yet babies and children, especially in the first few years of life, go to the doctor a lot more than most new parents realize. While your child's exact schedule may vary slightly depending on the practice, routine "well visits" typically follow a pretty standard timetable.

The first year is always the busiest. You can expect to see your pediatrician for the first time at three to five days after birth (though some may visit your child in hospital shortly after birth, followed by an in-office checkup a week later) and then at two weeks, one month, two months, four months, six months, nine months, and twelve months. Well visits slow down a bit in year two, going from every two to three months (approximately) to every three to six months. Expect to bring your kiddo in for a checkup at fifteen months, eighteen months, twenty-four months, thirty months, and thirty-six months. (After that, kids shift to an annual exam, just like adults.)

At each visit, expect your pediatrician to measure your baby's length and head circumference, as well as weigh your baby. Doctors use this data in two ways: to see where your kid falls on a standardized growth chart and to develop an individual chart that tracks your child's growth over time. When your doctor says, "Eduardo is in the 75th percentile for height," he or she is talking about where your child falls on those standardized charts, which describe weight for age, length for age, weight for length, and body mass index for age. For kids under two, these charts are based on data collected by the WHO in 2006, which, in its words, describe "the growth of healthy children in optimal conditions." After two years old, the charts are based on CDC data collected in periodic national surveys. The CDC charts were first implemented in 1977 and most recently revised in 2000. Unlike the WHO charts, these include all reported data from those national surveys, not just the data of children who met specific criteria. Both the WHO and CDC charts are available online, please see the Recommend Resources for more information.

Percentile charts rank *same-age kids* from lowest to highest weight, or shortest to tallest, and so on. However old you are, you're ranked against other kids the same age as you. So, if you're in the 75th percentile for height, like Eduardo, that would mean you're taller than 75 percent (or three in four) of other kids your same age, or that only 25 percent (or one in four) of kids your age are taller than you. With respect to percentiles, a big misconception I often hear in the office is that there's a problem if a child is on either the lower or higher end of a given chart. That's not usually true. Some people are just smaller or bigger than others. A kid might be short, and that is generally completely normal.

As a doctor, I'm looking to determine whether or not there is cause for concern, such as if a child falls at an extreme end of a growth chart (below the 5th percentile or above the 95th) and, very importantly, whether a child is following his or her own curve. For example, a child who is consistently at the 7th percentile for height but is growing and gaining weight appropriately at every visit, is likely just a small kid (parent stature is usually a pretty good clue to this as well). In contrast, a kid who is at the 70th percentile and then drops to the 5th percentile by the next visit would cause me concern. Such a child would have "fallen off" his or her own growth curve, signaling me to investigate further.

Beyond measuring your baby, the doctor will do a general exam, checking baby's skin, eyes, ears, throat; checking baby's reflexes, muscle tone, and strength; and checking to make sure all of baby's bits and pieces are in the right place. Then you and the doctor will speak. Some offices may have you fill out a questionnaire ahead of time. Either way, your doctor will check in with you to discuss baby's development. At every well visit, your doctor will touch on the upcoming milestones to watch for, as well as check in on the milestones baby should have attained by that point (fear not, we do a deep dive into understanding milestones and their timing starting on page 175 in the section called—wait for it—"Milestones"). You can review detailed charts of milestones for each age, and its corresponding well visit, on the CDC website (there's even a Milestone Tracker app and digital checklists available). Running through the appropriate list of milestones before a visit can be a good way to help organize any questions you might have about development. The opportunity to ask your pediatrician about anything that's been on your mind is probably one of the most invaluable parts of a well visit.

How to Get the Most Out of Your Well Visit

If you want to receive the best care possible for your child, the pediatrician–parent relationship should be a partnership. One of the best ways to be an active partner in your child's care is to arrive to well visits prepared. Come to your appointment with a written list of reasonable and appropriate questions—one that is, preferably, not thirty bullet points long. I can't stress this enough. When it's time to talk with your doctor, know what you want to chat about and run through your top concerns first.

Don't leave what's most important to you for last. At this point, I can't even count how many times a parent will have a question that he or she really wanted to address, but only first brought up on the way out the door. As I close my computer and turn to leave, "Oh yeah, one last thing . . ." It's usually the most pressing question and the one that takes the longest to answer. Unfortunately, doctors have only so much time. There's always another patient waiting, who also deserves to be seen on time and have full use of their allotted appointment slot. You don't want to have your important question rushed. Lead with it. Or at least raise it at the beginning of the discussion. "Oh by the way, my child was also having chest pain for the last three months," or "I was a bit nervous to say anything but I'm kind of worried Xavier might have autism. Thoughts?" are not the types of questions to ask when we are running low on time. If you have a major concern, please bring it up at the beginning so we can address it fully. I can't squeeze a chest pain discussion into one minute. Other helpful dos and don'ts for maximizing your well visit:

- Don't book a visit during your kiddo's nap time. This is a recipe for disaster and potentially many tears—not just your child's, but yours and maybe even mine.

- Don't bring more kids to a visit than you can manage. The visit won't go well with a nervous two-year-old on the exam table and hyper four-year-old twins bouncing off the walls whom you're constantly reprimanding, "Don't touch that!" We're happy to see your kids in back-to-back appointments for your convenience but be honest with yourself and consider whether or not this will actually work for your children, given their ages and temperaments.

- Ideally, make sure both parents (if there are two parents) can be at the visit. FYI, most practices are totally okay with having one parent there virtually. When both parents are equally involved in a child's care, there's no game of telephone, and the best decisions are made when both parties feel confident they have all the necessary information. Doctors do not have the time to call and update the parent that did not participate in the visit.

- Arrive on time to visits. Five minutes early is on time. We get that things happen. Your kid had a poop right before you left. There was a spill and you needed to change clothes. Trust me, we have heard it all. If your family is chronically late, please leave earlier. If your appointment is at 11:00, tell yourself it is at 10:45. I sometimes hear the excuse from parents that it is so hard to be on time because of the kids. Here is the thing to remember, us pediatricians *only* see kids. *Every one of our patients* are kids. Most of them somehow manage to be on time for their appointments. Yes, we need you to do your best to arrive on time because if everyone comes whenever they feel like it, the schedule will never work and it will negatively impact other families. Sure, we understand an unforeseeable event, such as a car accident or an emergency. It happens. Just please call to let us know you will be late. Don't just show up thirty minutes late. You have missed your whole appointment and are taking time from the next patient. I love when parents call to let us know they will be late. A simple "hi, there is a huge accident and we will be ten minutes late. Is that okay? Can you still see me?" goes a long way. If you're late once, we understand. However, I think I speak for every pediatrician out there when I say, don't be the chronically late family!

- Understand that doctors try their best to run on time. Sometimes, emergency appointments need to be squeezed in, complex kids may need more than their allotted time for new issues, or unexpected concerns might arise during a visit. As a result, the doctor may run late. You'd want us to see your child in an urgent situation, to take your child's mental health concerns seriously, or to spend a few more minutes with your family when you really need it, wouldn't you? So please cut us a break if we are running five minutes behind every now and again.

- Do recognize that, in response to most of your worries, your pediatrician will likely say: "It's normal." This doesn't mean your doctor doesn't take you seriously or is blasé. Most things are normal or simply need time to resolve. Also, situations progress and change; that is why communication with your doctor is so important. What seems like a basic virus at first may evolve over time with new or worsening symptoms and need to be reevaluated. Your doctor likely didn't miss your child's ear infection or pneumonia three days ago; it just hadn't progressed to that point yet.

- Do brag about your child. We love to hear about the awesome things going on in your kids' lives. Just you know, within reason, so we don't run too far behind for others.

- Do book your next appointment before you leave the current one.

- Do send a thank-you, compliment, photo, or toddler drawing our way, if you are so moved. It's not weird or "too much." We actually love it! Your doctor is literally there helping you keep your family healthy. A small gesture like a thank-you goes a long way in what can be a tough job. Most primary care doctors now take care of upwards of 2,000 patients. Outside your children's office visits, we mostly hear from families that are unhappy with billing, insurance, or other administrative issues, even though that is a mere 1 patient out of 1,000. We enjoy hearing from the other happy 999.

VACCINATION

For many people, vaccination has become an extremely emotionally charged topic—to say the least. I wish it didn't have to be that way. When it comes to vaccination, I believe the families I see every day are representative of most families in the US: they want to safeguard their children against childhood illnesses, support commonsense actions to prevent disease, prepare their children's bodies to fight infections, *and* understand what each vaccine is for, why it's given when, and what the risks may be. In other words, they want to be informed. As a doctor, informed choice is a cornerstone of my practice—it's what I believe is the right way to practice medicine. And that's my goal here: not to tell you what or what not to do, or when, but to arm you with the information you need to make informed choices. I support your right to choose what you feel is best for your child's health. I support vaccination and modern medicine. I support asking questions. I don't consider myself "pro" or "anti" anything, with the exception of being pro-parent and pro-child. This topic is close to my heart as I feel parents are sometimes unnecessarily shamed by the medical community for so much as asking questions.

The best person to have a vaccine discussion with is your child's doctor. In fact, if you have questions about any aspect of vaccination, you should address them during your search for a pediatrician.

What Are Vaccines and How Do They Work?

A vaccine is a preparation that helps train your immune system to recognize and fight certain pathogens, such as viruses and bacteria. Vaccines contain small amounts of inert, inactive, or weakened versions of the pathogens they're designed to fight. When introduced into the body—usually via injection (though sometimes orally or nasally)—the vaccine mimics an infection, stimulating the immune system to produce antibodies without causing the disease itself.

Think of vaccines like a blueprint for your body: if you later encounter a pathogen you've been vaccinated against, your body already knows how to produce the appropriate cells to fight it off. Vaccines can remain effective for anywhere from years to decades, and some, like the polio vaccine, may even provide immunity over the duration of your lifetime.

Current Vaccines

Since the introduction of the polio vaccine many decades ago, multiple vaccines have been approved for use in children. Every year, the CDC publishes a recommended immunization schedule for children that include the recommended age, number of doses, time period of each dose, precautions, and contraindications. Vaccines commonly given to babies and toddlers include:

- **Hepatitis B (Hep B):** Protects against the hepatitis B virus, which affects the liver
- **Diphtheria, Tetanus, Pertussis (DTaP):** A combination vaccine against three bacterial diseases—diphtheria, tetanus, and pertussis (whooping cough)
- **Haemophilus Influenzae Type b (Hib):** Targets bacterial meningitis and other infections caused by *Haemophilus influenzae* type b (this is not "the flu" even though it has a similar name)
- **Polio (IPV):** Protects against poliomyelitis, a viral disease that can cause paralysis
- **Pneumococcal (PCV13 and PCV15):** Protects against pneumococcal disease, which can lead to infections in the lungs, bloodstream, and brain
- **Rotavirus (RV):** Guards against rotavirus, a leading cause of severe diarrhea in young children

- **Measles, Mumps, Rubella (MMR):** A trivalent vaccine protecting against three viral infections—measles, mumps, and rubella
- **Varicella (VAR):** Targets chickenpox, a highly contagious viral infection

See the Recommended Resources section (page 249) for more information on CDC vaccine schedules.

Before your first vaccines are given, you should research and read up on the various vaccines available and recommended, weigh the benefits versus risks of each vaccine, and discuss your personal situation with your providers. By understanding the types of vaccines, the documented benefits, and their contraindications and risks, parents can make informed decisions about immunizing their children.

MILESTONES

Milestones are both a huge source of joy and anxiety. Early talking, early walking—early *anything*—parents will describe with pride in *full* detail, trust me. But if a kid doesn't hit a specific milestone at the average age—panic time. The thing is, very few of the parents wringing their hands over their kid's "late" start have children who are actually clinically delayed at something. What I see, over and over, both in my practice and online, is that most parents don't really know when to worry—or when *not* to worry—about milestones. In fact, the *whole idea* of milestones is often misunderstood, causing fear and unnecessary stress.

Yes, most doctors will reassure anxious parents that there is a wide range when it comes to normal for any given milestone and that each child is unique, advocating for a "watch and wait" approach. Admittedly, I say the same to parents all the time, but it's often clear the parent isn't convinced. Because what does "normal" even mean? And if the range is so wide (for example, it's generally considered normal for a child to utter his or her first word anywhere between ten and eighteen months), how do you know when your child's timeline *stops* being normal? *What are milestones even for?!* you might feel like shouting. Okay—deep breath.

A couple of years ago, I saw a set of eleven-month-old identical twins in my office. Their dads were concerned because one twin had started walking at ten months and the other was "only crawling." When one of the dads had first called, I tried to reassure him over the phone: "Walking at ten months is super early. That's wonderful that Milo is on the move already." He didn't seem to register my point. "Jasper isn't walking, though!" he insisted. The worried tone in his voice deepened and I adjusted course. Clearly, he didn't feel heard. "Bring them in and we'll take a look," I reassured him.

Two days later, there they were, the dads and the twins: Jasper, shy, nestled in his dad's lap, head buried in dad's armpit—as usual; Milo cautiously observant, eventually trying to grab at my stethoscope—as usual. Both boys showed normal muscle strength and tone (the amount of resistance to movement) when I checked them. I reviewed their histories: both had started sitting independently around six months. And when I'd last seen them, at nine months, they'd just begun to pull to standing and were crawling. All on track for them. Dad let me know that sometime since, Milo and Jasper had both started taking steps while holding on to a push toy. Except now . . . Milo was walking all by himself! Jasper was not! Cue the dread music!

Parents are always within their rights to worry. The thing is, both boys were healthy. Both boys had been meeting their milestones and making progress in their development—they were each continuing to gain new skills at a consistent rate. Jasper had not been sick in the past month, he hadn't experienced any physical traumas, and he hadn't displayed any other delays. In fact, he wasn't displaying a delay *now.* His brother was just moving a little faster than him. And come to think of it, his brother—who was born first (and will probably never let him forget it), had always moved just a little bit faster. He was a few days earlier on rolling and a week earlier on sitting. Nothing big enough to merit notice, or at least concern. But a month difference? For identical twins? Yep, still normal.

It's funny—of course, most first-time parents compare their child to other children. It's natural and normal, despite the reason there's a saying that "comparison is the thief of joy." Even when we tell ourselves not to, we compare kids. Usually, though, as new parents we compare our kids to extended family members' kids, friends' kids, coworkers' babies, or even to a scroll of kids we don't know, who fill our feeds and timelines via their "influencer" parents and their picture-perfect lives. But with Milo and Jasper, their dads had a built-in data set right at home. They had zoomed right ahead to the problem of second-time parents: comparing their own kids to each other. The problem is, even identical twins are far from identical. Even in infancy, Milo and Jasper had different personalities. And from the moment of their arrival, they had been doing things on slightly different but perfectly reasonable schedules. Yep, I'm about to say it: every child is unique. To put it in a way that is actually useful: *you should mainly focus on comparing your child against him or herself.*

Why "Average" Isn't Everything

"Okay, Dr. Joel," you might be thinking, "you just told us to only compare our child against him or herself. But what does that look like in practice? And what does it have to do with milestones? Worrying has become my natural state of being!" I got you. I mean, *yes,* other children and the average age at which they attain a milestone obviously provide the greater context we need when it comes to tracking development. But—and this is a big but—no kid follows the textbook exactly. Every kid moves at his or her own rate. Some do things faster than others and some do things slower than others. Some children may focus on one skill in favor of others. Babies and toddlers can be pretty single-minded, seriously. Just wait until you have to listen to "Let's Dance" by David Bowie for the millionth time in a single day. (Well, that may just be an Eli thing—he is much cooler than I'll ever be—but I promise you there *will* be a song or two on repeat for months that annoys the heck out of you.) A child might be on the later side of sitting independently, yet on the early side of cruising. Often, with specific skills (like stacking blocks or scribbling), it's family dependent. I see families all the time who might have a shelf full of Montessori toys but rarely do sensory play, or parents who spend a lot of time down on the floor playing, but aren't keen on process art. So, when I am gauging the appropriate development of a child in my office, I am worrying less about average milestone timing and focusing more on these three things:

- Progression: This is the *number-one* thing parents should focus on. Is your child making forward progress every month when it comes to overall development and milestones? If so, I'm not worried. For example, with rolling, I'm looking to see if your child is able to hold his or her head up when on his or her tummy. Is your child able to support his or her head without help? Can your child support his or her upper body with his or her arms when on the tummy? Has your child rolled from his or her tummy to back? If your child has hit the earlier milestones that support rolling, I'm not worried. If your child is not rolling from back to tummy yet, but is doing more than last time, I'm not worried. Even though your child might have arrived at the age where, on average, kids are rolling fully, your child is doing all the other things and has been moving forward normally. There are no other issues. Not worried.

- No Other Delays: Has your child had any other significant delays? This includes delays in domains other than the one about which you're worried. So, say you're concerned about a motor delay like walking—is your child delayed at any of the other age-appropriate milestones in the areas of social/emotional development, cognitive development, or language development? No? *And* you've been able to track your child's progress as above? Not worried.

- No Health Problems: Does your child have any chronic diseases or health issues? Has your child been hospitalized more than once? Does your child have frequent ear infections? Is he or she sick often? Is your child exhibiting any unusual physical issues, like favoring one leg or one hand? Are there any dysmorphic features? No, and your child has no other delays? You've been able to track your child's progress? Not worried.

As long as your child is progressing every visit and is growing, generally happy, eating well, and isn't at the threshold where it would be unusual not to be doing something (the age at which ≥75 percent are expected to do so), I'm not worried—and you shouldn't be either.

Of all the milestones, walking is one of the most variable. There is an approximate six-month range of when it usually starts (ten to sixteen months). By twelve months—the "average age" of first steps—only around 50 percent of babies are walking. That also means 50 percent are *not* walking.

Yes, I'm a pediatrician, not a mathematician, but according to my calculations, that's an equal amount of walkers vs. non-walkers. That means it's just as normal *not* to walk at twelve months as it is *to* walk. When it comes to "when to worry," the average age of walking is not the most information-rich statistic to lean on.

Of course, walking is one of the clearest, most concrete physical milestones children hit in the first two years of life. That's one of the reasons we're so focused on it as parents. Walking is also a perfect example of why, apart from health concerns, milestones mean so much to us. For parents, kids' milestones—especially the "biggies" like rolling, sitting, walking, and talking—are a sign not only of physical and cognitive development, but also of a child's growing independence (and possibly that we must be doing something right as parents). These types of milestones are big flashing neon indicators of the shift from helpless blob to that eventual teenager who'll be slamming the door in your face all too soon.

Of course, for many parents, hitting a milestone—or hitting one early—is confirmation that baby is a burgeoning genius. As a doctor, I don't consider a child hitting a milestone, whether early or on time, to be an achievement per se. As a parent, though, I witness my child's persistence and tenacity—and his surprise and joy—as he suddenly plops over on his tummy from his back or takes that first halting step, and I celebrate it. With Milo and Jasper, their dads were so consumed by their fear that they completely bypassed excitement and joy.

Look, there's absolutely no point in being worried about a kid that isn't walking at eleven months—it's an irrational fear. Ten to eleven months is really, really early to walk. As I spoke more with the twins' dads, I came to hear something else between the lines—the fear that *they*, as parents, had done something wrong. One kid was walking, so shouldn't the other one be too? After all, Milo and Jasper were identical twins! From my perspective, the twins were raised in the same home, at the same time, by the same people—and so their difference was likely not attributable to anything more than each child's innate human variability. Milo was two minutes older and already protective of his twin. He was the "scout" of the pair. In my opinion, Jasper would be right behind Milo momentarily, as soon as Jasper was sure the path was clear. Sure enough, a few days after their appointment, Jasper started walking with zero hesitation or stumbles.

Author and speaker Corrie ten Boom said: "Worry does not empty tomorrow of its sorrow. It empties today of its strength." In my experience, most worries are unnecessary. So consumed with the infinitesimal "what ifs," parents often miss out on the precious, fleeting moments that will never exist again.

More and more, I see parents in my practice missing out on moments of joy and excitement, of opportunities to celebrate their unique child's full potential. These parents appear so bogged down with guilt and anxiety because they are comparing their kids to other kids, and as a result, conclude their own children to be "lacking." Or, in the case of kids who hit milestones "early," parents equate their child's new skill with validation of their own parenting. Instead of being helpful guideposts on your child's development journey, milestones have instead become either a source of bragging rights (trust me, no one ever got into Harvard because they walked at ten months rather than thirteen) or an ominous marker laden with worry and fear.

The Difference Between "Could" and "Should"

Back in 2004, the CDC launched a new campaign, "Learn the Signs, Act Early," hoping to prevent parents from missing signs of potential developmental delays in kids who could benefit from early intervention. The campaign introduced a checklist of (drumroll, please) milestones, each tied to an average starting age.

Parents were meant to begin *actively* looking for the milestone behavior at its average age of initiation, in conversation with their doctor. The target age of any given milestone was meant to be a starting point, not a deadline. If a child had not met the milestone by the time *most* children had—defined as at the 75th percentile—then there might be cause for concern and further conversation with a doctor. Hence the traditional "watch and wait" approach.

The milestone markers were never meant as a *should*—they were meant as a *could.* Your child *could* begin walking by twelve months, because half of kids do. Yes, some kids might hit a milestone before the average age. After all, that 50 percent who begin walking by twelve months didn't all start simultaneously when the clock hit midnight on their first birthday. That fact has no bearing on the goal the CDC designed the milestone checklist to achieve: identification of *delays.* The 50th percentile marker was meant to identify a sort of tipping point. After it, the frequency of kids starting to roll, sit, walk—whatever the case may be—increases. And anywhere between that 50th and 75th percentile would still be considered on track, not late.

The problem is, over the next two decades, *could* morphed into *should* in the minds of most parents, creating a lot of stress, anxiety, and worry. Much of that was due to the problems inherent to the checklist itself—especially the use of the 50th percentile—as the CDC itself would eventually come to realize.

Much of that stress and anxiety has also been created—or at least exacerbated—by a comparison mindset nurtured by our friend, the internet. Two plus decades ago, when the CDC was getting "Learn the Signs, Act Early," off the ground, social media was in its infancy. Facebook was a Harvard student directory-meets-"Hot or Not" rip-off. Instagram was only a twinkle in a venture capitalist's eye. And blogs were primarily text.

Via one of the most popular types, the "mommy blog" (a "warts and all" peek into the stress, the mess, and the general chaos of parenting young children), parents began to "see" each other online and see what happened behind closed doors—*how* other kids were sleep trained, potty trained, fed . . . and *when* they hit certain milestones.

As the internet became more visual, the influencer was born: the mommy blog became more and more curated, a high-res platform for showing off a certain kind of life, one that was beautiful, organized, and centered around precocious children wearing adorable Pilgrim-chic outfits. (Okay, whether or not neutral linen baby bonnets are actually adorable is an argument for another time.) Little Aiden was toddling around at ten months; little Emma was practicing her letters with a beeswax crayon at two years old. Eventually, with the rise of apps, it became easier and easier for everyday people to share snapshots of their lives. These were rarely glimpses of their worst or even ordinary moments; they, too, were "curated." For those of us with kids, that meant those snapshots were (and are) generally posts of the "best" moments: notably, our children's "firsts"—first smiles, first words, first steps. When our own kids seemed to fall short, it became natural to worry. Social media introduced new pressures for parenting and childhood to look a certain way. Those *could*s kept snowballing into *should*s.

Meanwhile, after almost fifteen years of use and hearing from parents and pediatricians alike, the CDC came to see that there were some issues with the checklist in its existing form. So, in 2019, the CDC and the AAP convened a working group (a panel of subject matter experts) to revise the milestones checklist. Hurrah! In the AAP's own words, the goals of the group were to "clarify when most children can be expected to reach a milestone (to discourage a wait-and-see approach), and support clinical judgment regarding screening between recommended ages."

Finally, in 2022, after three years of work and almost twenty years after the first incarnation was launched, the CDC introduced the revised "Learn the Signs, Act Early" campaign. The biggest change is that milestones are now pegged to the 75th percentile instead of to the 50th.

When you look at the revised CDC milestones checklist, you'll see the language "What Most Babies Do by This Age" up top—that is, "What 75 Percent of Babies Do by This Age." This is *huge.* Going by the 75th percentile provides more clarity and less ambiguity for parents and caregivers about delays, removing much of the confusion between "could" and "should." If your child has not attained a milestone by the age cited on the updated checklist, then he or she may have a delay and may require intervention.

Unfortunately, this change was not met without controversy—it has been plagued, in particular, by the misguided idea that the CDC "lowered the bar" on milestones by moving many of them to later ages. Two things: first, the CDC did not announce new average ages of milestone attainment and, second, as we all now know, the old milestones, tied to the 50th percentile, were never designed to reflect, for example, when a child *should* be walking, only when that child likely *could.* In trying to truly home in on identifying delays and improving outcomes—the explicit goal of "Learn the Signs, Act Early" since its inception in 2004—the CDC shifted focus from an average age to the age that may begin to signal a delay. In other words, the CDC did not suddenly try to convince the public that the average age of walking is now fifteen months, no matter what you otherwise read on the internet.

DEVELOPMENT VS. DELAY

It's fair to say that most of us think of a milestone as a significant event that marks some kind of progress or change in our lives or in the world around us. And, yeah, no wonder—that is the definition of a milestone!

So, it makes sense that, historically, we've approached milestones as they apply to kids with this in mind. But with these big changes to the CDC checklists, it's clear now more than ever that we should really think of the new milestone guidelines as "When to Start to Worry"—instead of the general-interest "When Is the Average Age at Which I Should Expect My Kid to Do This?" most of us thought of them as.

In my practice, however, most parents are still interested in the average age they can expect their child to hit a milestone. I don't think that will ever go away. Curiosity about your child's development and excitement about "what comes next" are woven into the fabric of parenthood. While I stand by the fact that every child is unique and moves on his or her own timeline, I do encourage you to talk with your child's doctor at every visit about the normal range of development for same-age babies. Like most parents I see in my office, I wager most of you don't want to wait until your child reaches that bright red line at the 75th percentile to discover that he or she is experiencing a delay. Understanding the timeline between "average" and "delayed" can be a useful tool when considering whether or not a potential issue merits further investigation at that moment in time.

When should you worry about potential delays? As I said earlier, a single slow start in one arena doesn't automatically trigger my alarm bells. In identifying any potential delay, I'm looking for a confluence of factors—kind of like a puzzle. When I see a child in my office, whether it's for a well visit or because the child's parents are worried about his or her development, I grow concerned if I see any of these, particularly in combination with one another:

- No progression: Have your child's skills plateaued?
- Regression: Has your child lost skills or abilities they possessed previously?

- Other delays: Is your child currently, or has he or she been previously, significantly delayed at any other milestone, whether in the same domain or another domain?
- Health issues: Does your child have any ongoing health concerns, chronic illness, or hospitalizations?

While I'm a firm believer that most parents are worrying too much (and often about the wrong things), there are absolutely times when it is in the best interest of our child's health and well-being to involve a specialist who can dig deeper, rule out diagnoses, identify next steps, treat any issues, and support our kids in learning and practicing new skills. If you feel there is reason to worry and you're between appointments, don't wait for your next well visit. Make an appointment now to address this particular concern. Time is one thing we can't get back.

Bring notes to your appointment so that you don't forget anything. Discuss your concern in detail with your doctor. After your consultation, your doctor may refer you to specialists experienced in early interventions. These can include speech-language pathologists for verbal and swallowing issues; physical therapists for movement and bodily functions; occupational therapists for mastering daily activities; child neurologists for brain and nervous system concerns; and child psychologists or psychiatrists for mental and emotional well-being. A developmental pediatrician is also an option, particularly for children not developing at the same pace as their peers. By leveraging these specialists' expertise, you can better navigate the complex landscape of your child's needs.

The CDC is a great starting point for developmental milestones, but is not the end all be all when it comes to your child's development (and neither is any other single source). Their milestone checklists do not exactly spotlight what's developmentally important. Rather, they focus on how to identify delays, right? The two are related, yet also critically different. A great example of this is the CDC's removal of crawling as a milestone from the nine-month checklist. I didn't think much of this at the time. Although I certainly talk about crawling in the office around six to nine months and thought of it as an important milestone, I have never really considered it *essential.*

I've had several patients that never crawled and instead went straight to walking. They were otherwise healthy and exhibited no other developmental concerns. (Of course, it's hard to say if those children *truly* never crawled because I wasn't at home with them, but their parents stated as much.) If I had a patient who wasn't crawling at nine months, but was otherwise developing appropriately and had normal tone, I most likely would not refer that child to a specialist. If a child never crawled *and* didn't begin pulling to stand or walk at the appropriate age, that would be more concerning. Thus far, nothing in my experience has led me to worry about a child who is not crawling at nine months—and I don't think a parent should be concerned, either, if everything else is otherwise normal.

When I said as much in the newsletter I sent out after the CDC released its new milestones checklists, I was inundated with a flood of emails that surprised even me. (Trust me, I'm used to being on the butt end of dissenting opinions.) A number of therapists wrote back, emphatically opposed to the change, stating that crawling is essential for core body strength and brain development. Others responded by citing the ways crawling helps babies explore their environment, which is crucial to proprioception (your body's ability to sense movement and location). Many therapists suggested that if your child did or does go straight to walking, you should still work with them on crawling and help them master that skill. I think it's important to have humility and acknowledge that physical and occupational therapists most definitely know more about tone, motor skills, and fine movement and development concerns than I ever will. They do this every day. Yet, even after hearing from these therapists and exploring the issue further, I still would not necessarily refer a nine-month-old baby who isn't crawling to a specialist. I *would* now encourage parents to work on crawling with their child even if that child went straight to walking.

Given that the goal of the CDC milestone checklist is to identify delays, it can be true that crawling is both an important skill *and* doesn't have a place on the CDC milestones checklist. Like I said, there is little evidence that delayed or skipped crawling is a signal of a disorder or a precursor to negative outcomes. This does not negate its meaningfulness to a child's development.

Let me be clear: milestones checklists are not a screening, evaluation, or diagnostic tool. They are really a conversational tool. The truth is, there is not that much normative data on individual milestones. And that's okay. The bottom line is you know your child best. You know your child's moods, rhythms, and patterns. If you feel that anything is off, do not hesitate to speak with your doctor about it! If you are referred to a specialist or going through an early intervention program, know that there will likely be a wait. While you're waiting, one of the best things you can do with your child is just be truly present for him or her. Make time to put away your phone and play. Celebrate your child's unique capacities.

Celebrating All Our Kids

Our kids need us to see them, right now, as they are, rather than through the lens of an imagined ideal child that doesn't exist. On the flip side of parents like Milo's and Jasper's dads are the parents I encounter who get *validation* from their children's early attainment of milestones. We all want confirmation that our kids are secret geniuses. What I also know is that deep down, most of us want validation that *we* are good parents. We live in a culture that is sometimes not all that supportive of parents (for some there is no subsidized childcare, no paid leave, the list goes on), and yet, simultaneously, *there is so much pressure* put on parents. There's a "right" way to do everything these days, and it can be hard not to feel like you're missing the mark—especially when we're bombarded with images of other people's kids accomplishing x, y, or z. Finally, many of us live far from or don't have relationships with the family members, friends, or close-knit networks who might give us those emotional signals that we're not only not f*ing up, but we are also doing a damn good job. The Bubbe, Abuela, or Grandma who would invariably beam with pride, positively reinforcing our parenting skills, simply isn't around. Thus, it comes as no surprise that I see such an increasing number of parents who conflate the attainment of milestones with validation of their parenting. This is a lot to put on kids, especially kids who might hit their milestones later.

Definitely be excited and take pride in your child's growth—watching your kids attain skills and develop their personhood is among the most rewarding aspects of parenthood. At the same time, it's your job as a parent to be there to support your kid in the ways that will help him or her thrive. When your child takes his or her first step or first puts two words together, you should absolutely celebrate it. Your child is *supposed* to get there and yes, it's awesome when he or she does—just don't allow it to become the thing that *you* rely on to validate yourself as a person or parent.

I encourage you to keep an alternative milestones checklist, one that captures those intangibles and moments that you don't discuss at a doctor's office, but that nonetheless mark those unforgettable signposts on the road to shaping who your child becomes. Maybe your list will include the first time you played your baby your favorite song, the first time your baby heard your parent speak his or her native language, the first time your baby recognized a beloved relative, or the first time he or she tasted that dish that means "home" to you. Maybe it will be that day your baby no longer fits into his or her newborn clothes, the first time he or she dances, or the first time your baby calls someone a friend. Whatever it might be, it will be unique to your child—just as his or her milestone path is. Trust me—with your guidance, encouragement, and support, your child *will* get where he or she needs to go.

Language Development

One of our family friends loves to tell the story of her daughter's first sentence, spoken at eighteen months: "Mommy's coffee is hot." Apparently, she toddled down the stairs one morning and saw her mom holding a steaming cup. According to our friend, this was when she knew her daughter was exceptional—"She couldn't even see what was in the cup! She used deductive reasoning and abstract thinking!" Now let me add: our family friend is seventy-five and her daughter is forty-four. Over four decades have passed and this sentence is still a source of enduring pride for mom (and loving embarrassment for her adult daughter).

There is just something so incredibly affecting about hearing our children begin to speak. From the moment our children are born, many of us eagerly anticipate hearing their first words, no matter how good we are at relishing all their other aspects of development along the way. In my opinion, that's because language development is profoundly social and relational. Those first words, be they spoken or signed, are the building blocks of that first Mother's Day card, the car sing-alongs on the way to

Little League, the letter from summer camp, the call from the dorm, each and every "I love you" exchanged over a lifetime.

And of course, once children start using language, they are better able to communicate their needs—and we are better equipped to understand them. Though, at first, some of the toddler responses to your questions will leave you scratching your head. Once, at his request, I gave Eli some sliced apples for snack. Looking at the apples on his plate, he started crying. When I asked him what was wrong, he replied, "They're too slicey!" When kids begin using language they also begin developing one of the most unique and profoundly human aspects of their personality—how they communicate, how they express themselves, how they articulate their sense of the world.

Despite the stories our proud parents tell, how early or late we begin to speak doesn't strongly correlate with precocity or later success. We almost all learn to speak eventually. I would argue that what we really need to worry about is not *when* our kids start speaking, but how well we, as parents, support them in developing this skill. Focus less on what your child is doing and more on what *you* are doing to help your child communicate successfully over the course of his or her life.

LAYING A SOLID FOUNDATION FOR LANGUAGE

The fact is, the first three years of your child's life are the most intensive when it comes to acquiring speech and language skills. These skills develop most robustly in a language-rich environment—in other words, in an environment in which children are consistently exposed to the speech of other people. The big caveat here is that "the speech of other people" means the speech of other people *with whom they are interacting*. Babies learn best in a social context, meaning, a screen ain't gonna cut it. Yeah, yeah, yeah, we all know someone who has an eighteen-month-old that supposedly knows the alphabet from watching the child-entertainer-du-jour's videos on YouTube. That's not comprehension. That's rote memorization. Being able to chant "the ABCs" is not the same thing as being able to talk about the ABCs or understand what a letter is. There is no true interaction with a screen. (AI may very well change this in the future, but holograms are not the norm . . . yet.) A video may prompt a child to respond, but a video cannot truly respond to a child. There is no real organic interaction, the kind that best trains the brain when it comes to language. The bottom line is: you have to talk to your baby, a lot.

Let's face it, some of us are more naturally chatty than others. And talking to someone who can't talk back can feel pretty awkward (not to mention that polite society discourages us from monopolizing conversations). Some great ways to incorporate more speech into your everyday life with your child might look like this:

- Narrating Day-to-Day Activities: Simply tell your child what you're doing as you do it. Imagine your baby is an alien, or a time traveler from a pre-technological past. Explain how humans clean their clothes/the wonders of a washing machine. Why are you folding all those clothes up into neat little squares and stacking them into piles, anyway? Tell your child. Make it fun for yourself. Chat with your child about what you both see while out on a walk—the dogs you encounter, the flowers in bloom, you get it. Bonus: you start noticing the small details too. Honestly, this can really make life with a baby more enjoyable during what may otherwise feel like tedious moments.
- Narrating Care Activities: Use diaper changes, feedings, bath time, and the like to talk to your child about his or

her body. Explain what you're doing and why. Tell your child what's coming next and what to anticipate. Ask your child questions: "How does that feel?" "Oh, is the water refreshing?" "Is the plum sweet or sour?" It doesn't matter that he or she can't respond; you're helping your child learn about different modes of speech, helping him or her learn about things like intonation, and expressing care.

- Reading: It's never too early to start reading to children. Reading—as opposed to speech alone—exposes children to different sentence structures, aspects of language like rhyming and repetition, and words less frequently used in daily chat. In fact, a study from 2019 found that kids who read a single picture book every day are exposed to about 78,000 words a year. Doing the math here . . . if you read to your child every day between birth and age five, that's . . . a lot of words (390,000 to be exact) *just* from books. The researchers also found that in the years before kindergarten, children from literacy-rich homes cumulatively hear over 1.4 million more words than children who are never read to.

- Put Down Your Phone: This is not a guilt trip, I promise. (I could do better at this myself.) We all need to look at our phones sometimes—whether to send a text, order groceries, or just take a much-needed break. But one of the best ways to make room for more speech in your baby's life is to make more room in your own. If you're busy looking at your phone, you're not talking to your kid.

When it comes to *how* to talk to your baby, you've probably heard or been admonished not to use "baby talk." It is important that when we speak to our children that we speak clearly and use real words. But that might not mean what you think it means. Yes, you don't want to say, "Let me nibz that tootie-wootie," when you're telling your adorable baby you want to nibble his or her delicious toes. "Ooooh, I'm going to nibble that precious little foot" delivered in a singsong voice with lots of emphasis and exaggerated facial expressions? Go for it. That style of speech—emphasizing important words, speaking slowly, raising your pitch, and so on—is referred to very scientifically as "parentese." Not only is it nothing to be embarrassed of, it's actually universal across cultures and actively beneficial to your baby.

A 2022 study, the most wide-ranging study of its kind, analyzed over 1,600 voice recordings from more than 400 parents speaking to their infants. These parents were drawn from six continents, from diverse populations, and spoke eighteen different languages. The results of the study demonstrated that in every case, not only was the way parents spoke to their infants different from how they spoke to other adults, but also that the differences were markedly similar between all the parents—across cultures and across languages. A separate, earlier study—just one of many—found that the use of "parentese" in one-on-one interactions between parent and child correlated positively with language development. So, don't pay attention to the haters (who either don't have kids or aren't a lot of fun, anyway): go for all the silly faces, looooong vowels, and happy voices you want.

MANAGE YOUR EXPECTATIONS, WORRY LESS

Nine times out of ten, parents who come in to see me with concerns about a potential speech delay do not actually have a child showing signs of a speech delay. This is fantastic, obviously. And I'm always so happy to set worried parents at ease. What I have noticed is that many parents don't have a realistic understanding of when their child should be talking or, once the child starts talking, how much he or she should say at any given point. Almost universally, parents' expectations are way off the mark: too early and too much.

Parents also tend to focus too significantly and too early on expressive language, at the expense of paying attention to their baby's receptive language development. Speech (or signing)—that is, expressive language—is merely one component of using language. It helps to keep in mind that the word "language" really describes a system with shared rules that allows us to *communicate* with each other meaningfully. Children often have pretty advanced *receptive* language abilities—the ability to understand the meaning of speech—before they develop expressive language skills. They usually understand a lot of what you're saying before they can talk.

For a three-month-old, communication is going to look like crying to express a need, making noises and gurgling (this is the beginning of vocalization), turning their head toward a sound and/or startling at a loud noise (responding), and calming or smiling when spoken to, especially by their primary caregiver (recognition). Once the six-month well visit rolls around, I'm checking if baby is babbling, and if he or she is making some consonant sounds, like "p," "b," and "m." Does baby laugh? Does he or she look toward where a sound is coming from? Is baby responsive to a verbal change in tone from his or her caregiver? If you make a simple sound, will the baby imitate it?

It's really between seven months and a year where receptive language development comes into play much more fully—*and* where parents' expectations begin to get ahead of themselves. In these months, kids start developing an understanding of the world around them. Although they can't speak yet, they know the meaning of many words that are common in their life—words like eat, drink, cup, dog—and they may recognize the names of people in their immediate household (like "mama" or "dada" or a sibling's name). They start listening more actively and might be able to respond to simple requests ("Give me the spoon"). Their babbling becomes longer and more complicated—more like a mimicry of adult speech, with more consonant sounds. Eventually, they begin using expressive language in very simple ways, like saying "mama," and *using gestures.* We might not think of gestures as speech, but waving "hi" or "bye" or lifting the arms to be picked up is, indeed, expressive language.

Now, you may hear that at a year old, many kids say their first word. When I see a child at one, I'm not expecting him or her to talk. I want to know: Does the child understand some of what you say? Does the child make noises that sound like "mama" or "dada" (or something similar)? Does the child wave hello or goodbye? If the answer to any of those questions is yes, I'm not concerned about a child's language development, and you shouldn't be either.

Look, even the most advanced one-year-old I've met had only a few words max. And I've met plenty of one-year-olds, from many different backgrounds and with very different home lives. It's not until fifteen to twenty months that a child's vocabulary often expands to a dozen words or more. If my patient hasn't *tried* to say any words at fifteen to eighteen months, that may be cause for concern—the emphasis being on the word "try." I'm talking "ba" for "bottle" or "cah" for "cat." I don't expect any one-and-a-half year-old to have a large vocabulary, recite poetry, or use long sentences. I am looking for how well the child understands what's being said. Can he or she follow simple directions when gestures accompany verbal commands? Are the child's interactions with his or her environment becoming more complex—can he or she point to items when named? Is the child communicating what her or she needs—are you, the parent, better able to understand your child?

Before eighteen months, it is often just too hard to make a call regarding language delays based only on the number of words a child speaks. As a pediatrician, that's not what I'm focusing on. I am looking to see whether the child can hear. Does the child understand what's going on? Is he or she learning? Is the child moving forward and progressing? I'm not that worried about a child who knows what a lot of things are and is clearly following what's going on, but isn't saying much, as opposed to a child that doesn't seem to understand your requests and is not seemingly able to respond to what you're saying.

The "language explosion" really happens after eighteen months. It's pretty awesome to witness. Somewhere between eighteen and twenty-four months, most kids gain the ability to form simple two-word phrases, like "More milk" or "Dada up." They understand simple commands, like "Come here" without you needing to gesture. And they do learn—and love to use—at least one full sentence: "no" (an aspect of your child's speech you might come to wish was delayed). Your child's own gestures become richer—he or she might nod yes, blow a kiss, and, of course, point.

Once kids hit two years old, they are off to the races in what I like to call "The Little Linguist Olympics." During the year between two and three, kiddos sprout new words faster than they wipe their blueberry-stained fingers on your pristine white couch. It's as if one day they're saying, "Mama," and the next they're asking, "Are there aliens?"

Kids this age also have no filter. I can't tell you the amount of mortified parent looks in my office when their toddler answers a question in a weird way. I might ask, "What did you eat for breakfast, Anoosh?" to which he proudly replies, "Candy!" The embarrassed mother, who prides herself in feeding her child a wholesome, organic diet, quickly replies, "No you did not. You never eat candy." P.S. Parents, we know you did not feed your child candy for breakfast (probably). We enjoy the funny answers, and we don't judge.

Let me share another little tale. Timmy, two and a half, came in for his thirty-month well visit and proudly declared, "I poopoo!" His mom was flustered, but I was thrilled! "That's right, buddy, you did a poopoo, and that's amazing!" Why was I thrilled? Yes, a small part of it was his total lack of social graces. An even bigger part was his apparent pride. I love seeing a child relish his or her effort and consequent success. It's never too early to build healthy self-esteem. Perhaps the biggest reason for my excitement was the fact that Timmy was combining words to make a phrase—a sign that Timmy was right on track in his language development. Now, if by thirty months your tot is still at the "Me Tarzan, You Jane" stage of language, is speaking fewer than fifty words, or isn't using two-word phrases like "more water," then it might be time to ring the alarm bells (in the most holistic way, of course). Similarly, if your child's speech sounds like he or she is auditioning for the role of "Charlie Brown's Teacher" and is mostly unintelligible by thirty-six months, then we might need to delve deeper.

What causes language snags, you ask? It could be anything from chronic ear infections to not enough chitchat in a child's environment. Sometimes, an individual's brain wiring is just a bit different from the neurotypical, or there may be a family history of taking one's sweet time to speak. The American Speech-Language-Hearing Association has some fantastic guidelines on what to expect in these formative years—I encourage you to review their age-appropriate charts before well visits and make note of any questions that come up that you'll want to discuss with your child's doctor. (See Recommended Resources for further information.)

If you do suspect a delay, take a breath. The good news is that you're not just a spectator in the Little Linguist Olympics, you're a coach. There's no need to hit the panic button just yet; we have holistic options up our sleeves. First things first—talk to your pediatrician and get a thorough evaluation. Sometimes we'll recommend a consultation with a speech-language pathologist, the veritable language wizards of the medical world. These experts can offer targeted exercises that are essentially workouts for your child's vocal cords and brain connections.

Immerse your child in a rich language environment. Yes, that means more reading, storytelling, and pointing out things in nature during your weekend hikes—like "Look, a butterfly! Can you say butterfly?" Sometimes day care or preschool and being around other kids can encourage a child who can speak, but chooses not to. Nutritional support can also be crucial; omega-3 fatty acids aren't just good for the heart, they're brain food too! Sometimes, you have to nurture the soil to grow a beautiful flower—or, in this case, a burgeoning young linguist!

UNDERSTANDING AUTISM: RISING RATES, DEBATES, AND ENVIRONMENTAL FACTORS

Of all the developmental concerns, autism seems to be increasingly at the forefront for new parents over the last five to ten years. Perceived speech delays are often a catalyst for a parent to question whether his or her child may be autistic. All too often at the first sign of any new, mildly concerning behavior, a parent in my office will start asking questions about autism. I frequently remind parents that one atypical behavior, especially in the short term, is almost always normal. Kids will make all kinds of weird noises or have surprising movements, like a tongue thrust or a motor tic. Most go away within weeks after they begin. If a child is slightly behind in language, then that's worth discussing with your doctor, though autism should not be the first explanation that comes to your or your doctor's mind. If a child is shy, but otherwise communicative, makes eye contact, and has no other delays, I don't typically assume autism is the culprit.

Autism symptoms can manifest in a variety of ways and to varying degrees, which is the reason we describe autism as existing across a spectrum. Severe autism is characterized by profound challenges, including a marked lack of interest in others, limited eye contact, and a lack of emotional engagement. Repetitive behaviors are often highly pronounced, and there can be a notable restriction in activities and interests. In many cases, individuals may also experience sensory sensitivities and could have co-occurring conditions such as intellectual disability or epilepsy. The impact of these symptoms can be significant, often requiring intensive support and accommodations for the individual to navigate daily life.

There is no doubt that the prevalence of autism is on the rise. In 2023, the CDC reported a rate of 1 in 36 children, up from 1 in 54 in 2020. This is compared to 1 in 150 in 2000.

One of the ongoing debates about autism is whether its increasing occurrence is due to better diagnosis and awareness or whether autism is genuinely on the rise. While, in my professional opinion, I feel the rising rates of autism can be attributable to some combination of both, I also strongly believe autism rates are mainly rising because autism is more prevalent.

What is the underlying cause of this significant increase? At this point, we simply don't know. Some research links increased rates of autism with exposure to environmental toxins, advanced parental age, nutritional deficiencies, and genetic factors. Unfortunately, a lot more research is needed in this area.

Autism is, without a doubt, a complex and emotional topic the spurs some of the most heated debates. A deep dive into autism is outside the scope of this book—it is a book unto itself. From an integrative standpoint, a multifaceted approach that considers diet, environmental factors, and integrative therapies can play a beneficial role in supporting autistic children. In my opinion, focusing on the SEEDS, or foundations, of health (as described on page 3) is key to making the adjustments necessary to facilitate your child's resilience.

Early intervention and working with a variety of allied health professionals can be a game changer for children with autism, offering them tailored support to address developmental delays. Research has shown that early, targeted interventions can significantly improve cognitive and social skills, setting the stage for more positive long-term outcomes.

THE MODERN PARENT'S GUIDE TO SCREEN TIME

Ah, the dreaded topic—screen time. The AAP recommends zero screen time before the age of two, but let's be real. In a world where screens are ubiquitous, that guideline can feel not only unbelievably rigid, but shame-inducing for the many parents who don't follow it. Sure, some parents dismiss the guideline as deeply out of touch with modern life, while others feel conflicted—even guilty—for considering or allowing some screen time. In my mind, the question isn't necessarily whether the AAP's recommendation is right or wrong; it's about how to take an "ideal" scenario and adapt it for the real world. So, what does the science tell us about screen time? How does it affect your child's sleep and behavior? Are there ways to incorporate screens responsibly? Let's dig in.

The core concern with screen time isn't that watching *CoComelon* itself will turn your child's brain to mush (though it might jeopardize *your* sanity); it's that the time spent in front of a screen is time your child is not doing other, more beneficial and developmentally critical activities, like playing outdoors, talking with a parent, reading or being read to—you get the picture. Screens aren't inherently damaging, and we don't need to treat them like the bogeyman. What we do need to do is treat them as tools with specific uses, rather than use them as electronic babysitters. For instance, if you need a fifteen-minute break, screens can be a good way to let you recharge your batteries so that you can be a more attentive parent. Sometimes, a screen can be a better alternative to a meltdown in a restaurant or during a long car or airplane ride. In such scenarios, screens may be beneficial for both parents and kids alike.

When using screens responsibly, though, it's not only duration but content that matters. You should familiarize yourself with and monitor what your child watches. I'm no longer amazed by the two-year-old who can somehow navigate his or her way from an episode of *Bluey* on one streaming platform to what can only be described as mindless, foreign-country bot content on YouTube in fewer than seven seconds—because I've lost track of the number of kids I know who can and have done exactly this (my own included). And yes, while "educational" programs are better than a lot of what's out there, they are still typically much less effective than active, hands-on learning.

So, as long as your child is watching limited amounts of age-appropriate content, give yourself a break. If, maybe, you've been leaning a little heavily on screens, be honest with yourself, make a change, and most important, don't be hard on yourself. You haven't irreparably damaged your child, and guilt doesn't serve anyone. In fact, in my experience, most parents with whom I work experience guilt when it is completely unwarranted.

Take one of the families I work with: Tasha and Mike and their two-year-old son, Malik. Tasha had brought Malik in for his thirty-month well visit. When we got to the "screen time" part of the visit, she looked visibly anxious. "Dr. Gator, I feel awful about letting Malik have any screen time. I've read that it's bad for brain development, but I let him watch a little TV every night while I finish preparing dinner. I'm just not sure what to do." I offered a reassuring smile. Tasha had just finished telling me how she let Malik participate in cooking in whatever safe and fun way she could. Never mind that I knew this family had built a climbing wall just for their kids and that going to the library was their favorite Saturday outing. I gave Tasha my spiel about supervised, moderate screen time as a family tool—very much like what you just read. Tasha sighed in relief, "Thank you, Dr. Gator. You've really put my mind at ease." Now let me put your mind at ease: Screens are a part of our lives now. Watching a little TV is not going to set your child back. Watching a lot might.

However, one undeniable area of concern is around sleep and screens. The blue light emitted by screens has been shown to interfere with melatonin production, which is essential for sleep. For children who already have sleep issues, screen time near bedtime can exacerbate the problem. Avoid screens at least an hour before bedtime. There is a reason the last "S" in SEEDS is sleep. Protect it at all costs—or at least make sure the iPad stays out of the bedroom and out of the bedtime routine.

With Eli, we minimized screen time as much as possible. We certainly use screens, though. Screens have proven an invaluable tool at restaurants, on planes, or while traveling. My recommendation for screens is to use them responsibly, acknowledging their place in modern life, and making the best decisions for your family's individual needs.

Baby and Toddler Sleep

The first year of a child's life is marked by tremendous growth and change, not just physically but also neurologically and emotionally. During this crucial period, sleep plays a vital role in all facets of development. Infants, like newborns, continue to have erratic sleep patterns due to their underdeveloped circadian rhythms. Sleep cycles at this stage are much shorter than those of adults, and deep (or REM) sleep occupies a more significant proportion of sleep time. REM sleep is crucial for brain development, aiding in cognitive functions, memory consolidation, and emotional regulation. The American Academy of Sleep Medicine recommends that between four to eleven months, babies get about twelve to fifteen hours of sleep a day. Toddlers need between eleven and fourteen hours of sleep per twenty-four hours, including naps. Every child is different, though. I have taken care of perfectly healthy children who sleep more or less than average, but it's nice to have a range to shoot for.

Naps for toddlers can come in different forms: quick catnaps that last between twenty and thirty minutes, and more-restorative naps that extend for one to two hours. It's also okay if some days a nap doesn't happen; the key is to strive for a regular sleep schedule. Typically, toddlers may have a morning nap around nine o'clock or ten o'clock that can last from thirty minutes to one hour, and an afternoon nap, usually post-lunch, from about one o'clock to three o'clock that can extend from one to two hours. Eli dropped to one nap before he was two and was no longer napping as a three-year-old. We loved two to three hours of midday downtime on the weekends, so I was sad to see the nap go. Sarah, on the other hand, was in mourning. Ultimately, as nice as it was to have that break, life became easier after we were no longer forced to plan our weekends around Eli's nap schedule.

As toddlers grow older, they will naturally begin to phase out their daytime naps. Determining if a toddler is ready to drop a nap often involves keen observation of his or her sleep patterns and daytime behavior. Signs that your toddler may be ready to phase out a nap include consistent difficulty falling asleep during the usual naptime, waking up very early from naps, or showing extended periods of alertness and activity during the day without signs of fatigue. Another telling sign is that your toddler sleeps well at night even when a daytime nap is skipped. Once you recognize these signs, the transition away from napping can be gradual. Start by allowing your toddler some quiet time; if your toddler doesn't fall asleep within a reasonable amount of time, let him or her come back to play. Then skip that nap every other day, increasingly extending the days between naps until nap time is phased out completely. As you make these changes, be sure to monitor your child's nighttime sleep and overall mood to ensure he or she is still getting the rest needed. For us, we knew naps were coming to an end when Eli began fighting them. At first, it was random: some days he would nap and others he would not. He would call to us after a few minutes that he was "done sleeping." He would lay there, looking at books or playing instead of napping. After this happened off and on for a few weeks and then for three consecutive days, we gave up. Generously put, he was not the best version of himself in the week that followed. After a week, and a slightly earlier bed time, he seemed to adjust to his new sleep schedule.

Sleep regressions are another common phenomenon during infancy and toddlerhood. They are periods when a child, who had been sleeping relatively well, suddenly starts having issues with sleep, such as frequent awakenings, difficulty in falling asleep, or changes in sleep patterns. Typical ages for sleep regressions include four to six months, eight to ten months, eighteen months, and again at around two years. They seem particularly cruel when you have just grown accustomed to sleeping through the night again for the first time since the birth of your baby. The key to navigating a sleep regression is patience, as these are generally phases that will pass. It's also beneficial to maintain a consistent bedtime routine to help your baby or toddler through this time. If a sleep regression seems to be adversely affecting your child's health or behavior, talk to your pediatrician.

When it comes to transitioning to a toddler bed, the appropriate age varies. Typically, it happens between eighteen months and four years. Signs that your toddler may be ready for this transition include climbing out of the crib, asking for a "big-kid bed," or showing signs of potty-training readiness. The transition itself should be managed carefully to ensure it's a positive experience for your child. Introduce the new bed as an exciting change. If the bed is high off the ground, implement safety measures, such as guardrails. Maintaining a consistent bedtime routine during this period can also go a long way in helping your child adapt to a new sleeping environment.

SLEEP TRAINING

Sleep training is the process of helping a baby learn to fall asleep—and stay asleep—independently. There are a number of different approaches from "Cry It Out" (also called the "Extinction" method) to Bedtime Fading and the Ferber Method (also called "Check and Console"), among others. Which method to choose depends on your parenting style and comfort level with crying, though most parents I work with find the Ferber Method to be a happy middle ground. This method, developed by Dr. Richard Ferber (a pediatrician and the director of the Center for Pediatric Sleep Disorders at Boston Children's Hospital), involves letting your child cry for a set period of time before checking on him or her, then progressively increasing the time between checks, until your child falls asleep. This teaches baby to self-soothe while still feeling secure. Regardless of which method you choose, consistency is essential for successful sleep training. A consistent bedtime routine, timing, and approach can make the process smoother and more effective for both child and parent.

Whether or not to sleep train can be a controversial topic among modern parents. Many parents fear that sleep training could emotionally scar a child. Yes, your baby may (nay, *will*) cry. But numerous studies have shown no long-term negative effects on the child's emotional or psychological well-being from sleep training. In my opinion, sleep training, when done correctly, is not a heartless act, but a thoughtful, considered process that can benefit the entire family. As with many things in parenting, teaching a child something new may be frustrating for both parent and child, for a short time. That fleeting frustration is typically forgotten by morning, replaced with a bright smile.

Some people do not believe in sleep training. If you fall into this category, I respect your decision to do what you feel is best for your child. In general, I think the choice to sleep train falls in the realm of "do it if you feel comfortable, when you feel comfortable, and if it is in line with your values."

Personally, in my years of experience, families getting longer stretches of sleep are much happier and well rested. Some parents, influencers, and professionals say you can't train a baby to sleep, yet there is a whole industry devoted to it. And based on seeing parents who are exhausted before sleep training and refreshed one week later after sleep training, I can confidently say that you can teach, train, support (or whatever word you want to use) your baby to sleep for longer stretches. When considering the pros and cons of sleep training, I encourage parents to focus on the process itself to determine if it makes sense for them. Some pros and cons to consider include:

Pros

- Better Sleep for the Family: When a child can sleep independently, everyone in the family typically gets more restful sleep.
- Life Skills: Sleep is a life skill, and teaching children to self-soothe and sleep on their own can promote independence and emotional regulation.
- Parental Benefits: Especially in households where both parents work, a solid sleep schedule can be beneficial for managing stress and daily responsibilities.

Cons

- Initial Stress: The early days of sleep training can be emotionally tough for the parents as well as the child.
- Inconsistencies: Life events, like illnesses or traveling, can disrupt sleep schedules, requiring a "retraining" period.
- Not One-Size-Fits-All: Some children may not respond well to certain sleep training methods, necessitating trial and error.

Remember, whatever method you choose, the major parenting goal for sleep is to help your child develop healthy sleep habits. Numerous parents in my practice never sleep trained, and their children learned to sleep wonderfully on their own. Even for "high-needs babies," many families I have worked with have found healthy and safe ways to get enough rest without ever having to do anything that includes "crying or training." For those that do ultimately decide that sleep training is for them, experts that support sleep training differ on their recommendation for when to begin. Most feel it can be appropriate to start sleep training between four and six months (although, in my experience most parents choose to sleep train closer to nine months to one year).

No parent has ever told me they regretted sleep training. Most wish they had implemented it sooner. Not only are the parents better rested, but more important, baby is better rested. Parents teach their children other essential life skills from a young age, such as feeding, using the potty, and so many others. If parents can train and support their children through these other tasks, sleep should not be an exception. Sleep support helps lay the foundation for a lifetime of healthy bedtime habits.

Independence

Welcome to the section on toddler independence, a topic that touches the hearts and tries the patience of parents everywhere. As your little one takes his or her first steps into the world—literally and metaphorically—your child is laying the groundwork for his or her own autonomy. With this newfound independence comes inevitable challenges: the stubborn refusals, the impassioned tantrums, the highly debated topic of discipline, the often-bewildering phase of potty training, and the natural but sometimes uncomfortable period of body exploration. It's a whirlwind journey, yet one that holds invaluable lessons for both you and your child. In this section, we will delve into these nuanced issues with a balanced perspective, empowering you to guide your toddler through this exciting, albeit often tumultuous stage—all while honoring your child's unique developmental path.

TODDLER BEHAVIOR

The "terrible twos" is a term that has become synonymous with toddlerhood. While there can be something almost tyrannical, something very

Napoleonic, about toddlers that's sort of adorable (when they're not currently terrorizing *you*), I'm not a fan of this terminology. I don't like attaching negative verbiage to normal child behavior. We might not like it, but that doesn't make it bad. Perhaps my biggest issue with this phrase is that it's misleading: most parents start seeing "terrible twos" behavior while their child is still one—often around fifteen months.

It makes sense when you consider that a baby's first steps—tottering, teetering . . . you know, *toddling*—are the most literal marker of early toddlerhood, a phase of life that is all about a child's growing independence and assertion of self. Crawling and then walking are, in many ways, a child's first self-directed separation from mom and dad. The years between one and three mark a whirlwind of developmental leaps. During this time, kids go through major transformations of their social, emotional, and cognitive faculties. These changes can be kind of misleading for parents—suddenly, our kids seem so much older! They have opinions! They can have conversations! It's all too easy to forget they're not mini adults (we're still changing their diapers). Their brains are not like ours, quite literally. They are still developing. Much of what we take for granted, like emotional regulation, they're simply not fully wired for yet (though I know plenty of grown-ups who don't seem wired for it, either). And when you combine a still-developing brain, new skills, and a strong need for independence, the result can be behaviors that many parents find puzzling to say the least. Challenging, too—though that's the polite word for it. There is a reason an entire industry of toddler-whispering books, courses, podcasts, and social platforms exists.

And we're lucky to live in a world where that "industry" is thriving. There are so many fantastic experts out there with solid, actionable advice that can be truly transformative for parents (see the Recommended Resources section for some of my favorites). However, I find that even knowing where to start, when it comes to everything out there, can be overwhelming for the parents I see who are mired in a toddler rough patch. Yes, I point them to the same resources you'll find at the end of this book. But for the parents in my practice, it really helps them feel less frustration (and actually pick up a behavior-focused book or sign up for an online course) when they remember, first and foremost, that their toddler's behavior—even when, *especially when*, it is trying—is not personal (your toddler isn't enacting a tiny-sized personal vendetta against you), and, for the most part, can't be helped.

Toddlers are *going through it.* Seriously. The key to really "getting" them is understanding how much work they are doing to become a person (more than many adults in therapy). Toddlers are engaged in a daily battle between their struggle for independence and their ongoing attachment to their family. They're just developing impulse control. *And* they're trying to make sense of the world that their new skills are opening up to them. This is a lot for any human to manage, especially simultaneously. All of this shows up in an array of "hallmark" toddler emotions and actions.

Curiosity: Toddlers want to touch, taste, and explore everything around them. This is their way of discovering and learning about the world. While this is crucial for cognitive development, it also means they can create havoc and get into situations that might be unsafe. They don't really grasp true cause-and-effect and aren't capable in the same way an adult is of thinking-before-acting. The challenge for parents is to help them take *appropriate* risks (getting a few bumps and bruises jumping around the playground is overall a good thing)—encouraging, not stifling, their inquisitiveness, while keeping them from real harm. Part of this means setting up an environment that is conducive not only to their explorations, but also to your patience with their explorations. I see a lot of parents who are frustrated that their toddler is "always getting into things" and "doesn't listen." Look, a toddler does not "know" at first that the vase is breakable, that it's special to you, or that they shouldn't touch it. If you leave it on your low-to-the-ground mid-century coffee table and your toddler accidentally knocks it over, it's on you to control your emotions. They were not careless—you were. Remember that their need to explore and their curiosity drives much of their behavior. If there is a sharp corner on your table and the table is right beside your couch, you can rest assured they are going to jump off that couch like a trampoline at some point and bang into the table. Move the table out of the head-banging radius to prevent the ER visit. Sarah continues to scoff at me for continuously mucking up her home aesthetics (she should be an interior designer; seriously it's impressive, and I ruin it), but Eli's head has thanked me on more than one occasion. They are going to jump. They are going to dive headfirst off your bed. They are going to touch and knock over everything. This I can promise you, so be prepared and move it out of their reach.

Asserting autonomy: As toddlers begin to see themselves as separate entities from their caregivers, they start asserting their will. Phrases like "I do it" become common, signifying their desire to take control. This can also manifest as what adults perceive as "defiance." The popular toddler sentence "No!" is not about defiance, though. Saying "no" is a toddler's way of testing boundaries and limits, understanding decision making, and reinforcing their sense of self. Often, it's also their safety net, shielding them from the unfamiliar and keeping them within their comfort zones. While caregivers should respect and understand this newfound assertiveness, not every declaration of "no" can or should be entertained, especially concerning safety. Honestly, the hardest part of my parenting journey so far has been teaching Eli to swim. The fountain of tears, the parade of nos, has been heartbreaking. Putting his head under water was one of the most drawn-out, terrifying things for him. And with good reason. It is scary to swim—you have no control, and you can't breathe under there. I get that. But it is important. His grandparents have a pool in their backyard, and I know it is possible he could fall in. If I listened only to his words, he still would not be swimming. Instead, I pushed him through the fear, and after putting on his goggles and finally going under the water just once, he proudly stated that putting his head under water was his "favorite thing." Offering structured choices and reinforcing positive behaviors can guide toddlers toward more constructive expressions of their independence.

Imitation: Toddlers learn a lot by mimicking adults. It's not uncommon to see them pretend-playing with phones, pretending to cook, or even mimicking daily chores. This is a constructive way they make sense of the world around them.

TODDLER DISCIPLINE

Over and over, parents tell me that learning their toddler's "challenging" behaviors are normal makes it easier for them to manage those behaviors. Most important, it makes it easier to manage *their own responses* to the behaviors—and that's what tends to make the biggest difference when it comes to easing parental stress. That's because it really is *your* mindset—*your* attitude about and approach to managing the vagaries of toddlers' moods—that is responsible for a large part of the friction that comes with this phase. Once you know what's ultimately behind your toddler's actions—even if the immediate "reason" remains a mystery—it becomes easier to embrace shifting to a proactive rather than reactive mindset. By shifting how you *think* about toddler behavior, rather than hyper focusing on what to *do* about toddler behavior, you set yourself up for success. With parents in my practice, when it comes to mindset, we talk about the need to:

Align your expectations with reality. Toddlers do not behave like grown-ups because toddlers do not think like grown-ups. Trying to reason with them using adult logic is often not helpful—so I don't suggest you do so. If you do, don't expect them to respond to it productively. And you should refrain from getting upset when they don't.

Stop thinking of behaviors as good or bad. Toddlers do what they are designed to do, which is learn about the world and how to be in it. You might not like a behavior, you might find a behavior challenging, and a behavior may even be dangerous or antisocial, but that still does not make it "bad." Your role as a parent is to help your child learn how to regulate and express his or her emotions, feel and *be* safe, understand societal norms, and develop healthy interpersonal relationships—over time. Focus on these goals as you course correct certain behaviors and reinforce others. Remember, the root of "discipline" is the Latin *disciplina*, which literally means "to instruct" or "educate," not "to punish."

Accept annoyance. Here's the deal: not all behavior you personally dislike needs to be "corrected." Sure, you set the ground rules in your home. If they drive you insane, don't buy loud, blinking toys. In such a case, buying a fire truck with a button that plays a "realistic" siren noise is a recipe for disaster. I guarantee your toddler will press that button every two minutes. (Eli sure did. Somehow the siren "stopped working" the day after he received that present. The batteries were definitely not removed—wink wink.) Pressing the button on a toy every few minutes may be annoying behavior to you, so it makes sense to bypass the frustration. Despite your best efforts, your child will learn a song you despise or a silly noise he or she will repeat over and over. It's important your child feels not only that you love him or her unconditionally, but that you like him or her. Resist setting up a dynamic where you're essentially normalizing "criticizing" your child for developmentally appropriate behaviors.

PARENTING STYLES

Parenting a toddler can be like navigating a ship through turbulent waters. The unpredictability and mood swings can catch even the most prepared parents off guard. Maintaining a balance between gentle guidance and firm boundaries—without veering into the permissiveness that is often attributed to gentle parenting—is central to effective toddler parenting.

Back in the 1960s, renowned developmental psychologist Diana Baumrind identified and defined the three primary parenting styles as authoritarian, permissive, and authoritative. Later, in the 1980s, psychologists and researchers at Stanford Eleanor Maccoby and John Martin would add a fourth: uninvolved. Their work is still acknowledged today as foundational to understanding parenting.

The authoritarian style is high on demands but low on responsiveness, leading to children who might be obedient but also suffer from low self-esteem. The permissive style, conversely, is high on responsiveness but low on demands, often resulting in children who lack self-discipline. Uninvolved parenting is low on both demands and responsiveness. Authoritative parenting strikes a balance, being both demanding and responsive. Research has consistently shown that children raised by authoritative parents are more likely to become independent, self-reliant, and socially accepted individuals.

Many of our parents and grandparents employed the authoritarian "my way or the highway" style of parenting—that all-too-familiar "just wait till your dad gets home" or "don't make me pull this car over." The rise of permissive parenting can be seen as a pendulum swing away from the authoritarian parenting style that dominated previous generations, creating a shift in recent years to a "gentler" approach to parenting.

Rooted in the desire to respect children as individuals with their own thoughts, feelings, and needs, gentle parenting has aimed to create a more egalitarian family structure. However, like any pendulum that swings too far in one direction, there's a risk of unintended consequences. In the pursuit of a "better" approach, some parents have inadvertently tipped the balance into permissiveness, blurring essential boundaries and diluting the importance of consistent, developmentally appropriate consequences. This ultra-lenient parenting can confuse children and create an unstable environment that lacks the structure kids need for healthy emotional development. Thus, while the intentions behind gentle parenting are commendable, its application requires a nuanced balance to ensure that children are both respected and guided.

Here is the way I reinforce this point to families in my practice. Imagine you are in a car at night driving over a bridge in very low light. If there are no guardrails, you will have to drive really, really slowly so you don't fall off the side. If, however, there is a large wall on each side, you can drive a little faster since you will be less worried about falling over the edge. Toddlers work like this. They thrive with reasonable boundaries. They are going to bang against the walls at times, but they can move forward a lot faster if they know where those guardrails are. Having appropriate boundaries does not stifle their development. It in fact lets them develop faster. They 100 percent need appropriate boundaries to learn, and if you are doing a gentle parenting course that tells you anything other than that, close your computer.

You are the adult. You are teaching them societal norms. They don't know it isn't appropriate to pee on your living room rug. They don't know you need to get up for work tomorrow morning, so they can't have a snack at two in the morning. While it's essential to be mindful of a child's feelings and needs, a complete absence of rules and consequences will lead to challenges both at home and in broader social contexts. Lack of rules leads to the entitled "Santa Monica" free-range children I see all too often, running amok with reckless abandon. For example, you can easily spot them at any number of local restaurants, racing around the tables, screaming and throwing things, while their parents sit just feet away, looking self-congratulatory and ignoring the chaos. Have you noticed the growing prevalence of hotels that have gone kid-free? Why do you think that is? Maybe they know that some parents cannot be trusted to set appropriate boundaries for their children, who disturb the other guests. When we travel with Eli, we are limited by where we can stay in Palm Springs because every hotel seems to have gone in that direction. And I don't blame them. But I do hope we can change course and raise the next generation of children with appropriate boundaries.

Consistency in implementing boundaries is equally important to avoid sending mixed messages to your child. Being attuned to your child's emotions and needs and setting firm boundaries and consistent consequences are not mutually exclusive propositions. In setting firm boundaries and consistently implementing consequences, you teach your child not just to respect others, but also the norms and rules that will ultimately help him or her become a socially competent adult. By understanding the research and acknowledging the complexities of toddler behavior, parents can take steps to be both "gentle" and "firm" caregivers. Remember, the research shows that authoritative parenting leads to the most well-adjusted children. Your love, understanding, and consistent boundaries will set the stage for your child's emotional and social success.

TANTRUMS

Ah, tantrums. Understandably, most parents dread tantrums. Few things test our parenting patience more, especially when they happen in public or at time-sensitive moments. There's little that can trigger a stress response more quickly than your toddler screaming in the aisles of Target or resisting being buckled into their car seat on the way to day care (while you are already late for work). Characterized by crying, screaming, resisting comfort, and even aggressive behavior, tantrums are emotional outbursts that are *a response to unmet needs or desires.*

To us, a child might seem like he or she is having a tantrum "for no reason" or simply because that child is not getting what he or she wants (which we tend to view with disapproval). That's not the case. It's critical to understand that tantrums are not just a product of a child's whims. They are the child's way of expressing a frustration that he or she may not understand and/or can't articulate. At this age, toddlers are navigating a world bustling with new challenges, rules, and expectations. Their limited language skills compound their difficulties. Imagine the exasperation, anger, and sadness you'd feel if you needed something and no one could understand you.

Before the Storm: Strategies to Preempt Toddler Tantrums

Given that tantrums are typically the by-product of an unmet need, one of the most effective ways to deal with tantrums is to do your best to preempt them. Physiological factors such as fatigue, overstimulation, or hunger can precipitate tantrums—being "hangry" is real. Toddlers, in their early stages, are still acquainting themselves with emotional regulation. The simplest deviations, like missing a nap or being overwhelmed by the sensory overload of a busy place, can make them more susceptible to emotional meltdowns. Their environment, particularly unfamiliar or restrictive settings, can add another layer of complexity, making toddlers feel overwhelmed or confined, leading them to throw tantrums as a way to reassert control over their surroundings. Maintaining consistent routines, safeguarding naps, allowing adequate big body play (i.e., getting enough active time), ensuring timely meals, and facilitating adequate rest can forestall many common tantrum triggers. I know that might sound obvious. Truly, though, our own lives are so busy and so hectic that providing this kind of consistency can be not only hard to do, but easy to miss as the problem. Kids, toddlers especially, thrive off routine and structure. Knowing what to expect gives them security, which can make them feel more in control and less stressed. Learn your child's needs and anticipate them.

Managing the Meltdown: A Calm Approach to Toddler Tantrums

Addressing tantrums often requires a nuanced approach, blending empathy with firmness. Start by ensuring your child's safety. Then acknowledge his or her feelings. Simply recognizing a toddler's emotions and validating them can sometimes be all that's needed to alleviate his or her distress. Talk to your kiddo. Just don't try to reason with a toddler or use adult logic to persuade him or her that he or she shouldn't be upset. Your goal in conversation is to discern your toddler's needs, not interrogate him or her for a "reason." Strategies like distraction, redirection, or even offering them limited but acceptable choices can often defuse tense situations. No matter what, it's paramount that you maintain your composure. If you can't, make sure your toddler is safe and step away for a minute, letting him or her know—kindly—that you are taking a breath, or whatever, to help calm yourself down. Never make your response your toddler's responsibility. Telling a toddler "You're upsetting me!" or "You're making me angry!" teaches it's not okay to express emotions. When you stay calm, you not only model desirable behavior and emotional regulation, but you also don't add fuel to the tantrum fire. Reacting aggressively or with heightened emotions will only intensify the situation. Be your toddler's rock.

Tantrums are often the biggest concern of parents of toddlers. I do remind parents who are near their breaking point that tantrums are normal and that this is just a phase. When they're in college, your children will not continue to drop to the floor, banging their legs, arms, and head because they didn't get the cookie. Just a few quick decades and the tantrums are sure to resolve on their own, so hang in there.

Potty Training

During the last few minutes of my patient Ethan's two-year well visit, his mom, Stephanie, mentioned that she was feeling very anxious about potty training him. I thought Stephanie meant she was nervous about beginning the process—completely understandable. Stephanie quickly clarified that they were in the midst of potty training and, in her words, Ethan wasn't "getting it." She had read a number of books on the subject and tried at least three different methods. The last book Stephanie had read stated that if potty training doesn't happen by thirty months, parents will have missed the ideal window, making the whole process immensely more difficult. (What?!)

As Stephanie talked, she swung between criticizing herself and worrying that something might be wrong with her two-year-old. I asked Stephanie why she and her husband had decided to start potty training in the first place. "Well . . . almost all my friends who have kids Ethan's age have potty trained," she said. "And in a couple of months he's starting at a preschool that requires it." Wanting to better understand Stephanie's anxiety about Ethan himself, I asked her for more detail about his response to potty training. "First, he just seems totally uninterested. My husband and I talked to him about picking out his own potty and decorating it with stickers and he wasn't excited at all. We told him he could get big-boy undies with superheroes, and he didn't care. Second, whenever we try to make him sit on the potty, he resists. And he gets really upset if we tell him he can't wear a diaper and shouts 'No! I keep my diaper!'" Stephanie raised her eyebrows, looking at me with an expression like, "Something is wrong with him, right?" Everything Stephanie shared with me only confirmed that Ethan was a perfectly normal toddler—one who maybe wasn't quite ready for potty training.

Stephanie is far from alone in believing that there's an ideal time to potty train (or that missing that window of opportunity spells disaster). The number-one question parents ask me about potty training is *when* to do it—quickly followed by asking when is "too late." Here's the thing: there is little scientific evidence that supports the benefits of one potty-training method versus another, or that includes timing. Accepted norms around potty training are more about cultural values. It's true that children in other countries may train earlier overall than in the US, and it's also true that in the US, people used to train earlier than they do now. But in all those cases, the norms are still ultimately very much about parental values and needs, rather than an explicit physiological or developmental requirement on the part of kids. Diapering is expensive, dirty diapers are inherently kind of gross, and most parents don't like changing them. There's an undeniable ick factor and an element of inconvenience at play—for parents. And as far as what folks did back in the day, having to rely on old-school cloth diapers (messier, extra laundry, not as absorbent, etc.) probably provided a greater push to get children out of them sooner.

Parents often feel societal pressure to potty train their children early. I encourage you to question whether the rush to potty train is really for your child's benefit or due to external pressures. Personally, as a pediatrician, I feel that the generally appropriate window for potty training is reasonably wide: from one and a half to four years old or so. In thinking about when to potty train your child, it's not about a "should." It's about *your child's* readiness. That's the key factor in determining when to start.

Every child is unique and will be ready for potty training at his or her own pace. The age to start can vary significantly from child to child. There are some basic abilities all kids need to start potty training, of course: They need to be able to learn to recognize when they're about to pee or poop—this isn't really possible developmentally until after eighteen months. They must be able to understand basic instructions and follow them. They need to be able to pull their bottoms down and pull them back up (with a little help is fine). In my experience with countless kids, given those abilities are in place, children will potty train when they're ready—you just need to watch for those signs of readiness. What do they tend to look like?

Signs your child may be ready for potty training include showing interest in toilet use, indicating a dirty diaper either verbally or nonverbally, staying dry for extended periods, and expressing social awareness about toileting. These cues hint at both physiological and psychological readiness, making it an optimal time to introduce potty training.

If you do have to train for preschool, because of other external factors, or because you want your child to learn, then just do it. Prepare yourself, set your life up so you are able to deal with your child's accidents for at least several weeks, take his or her diapers off, and dive in. Be consistent. If you are steadfast on teaching your child at two years, you can most likely do so if you are consistent. For some children, it may be a whole lot easier at three. For other kids, two and a half is the perfect age. If your child simply isn't ready, and the school requires it, that may not be the best school for your child. There are many schools and care centers that do not require children to be potty trained to enroll and that support parents in training their child when the child is ready; I would recommend you consider this when thinking about a good fit for your child.

Personally, I have never understood what all the rush is about. Using a diaper is so much easier than trying to find a bathroom every hour or two, especially when in the car or traveling. I am confident we could have started potty training Eli earlier, but we had no interest in a struggle. My wife and I waited until he was about three. We were going on a major international trip and decided it made more sense to start potty training after we returned. We were concerned about being able to make it to the bathroom quickly and regularly enough in airports and on the plane, and about finding bathrooms while abroad, especially since we were not fluent speakers of the local language. We told Eli when we returned there would be no more diapers during the day. The day after we got back, we stuck to our word. He moaned and groaned for an hour or two (typical Eli). He was going on the toilet later that same morning. With the exception of a few minor ups and downs, he was out of daytime diapers and going on the potty within a day. Of course, there was still the occasional accident, but honestly—and I attribute this to the fact that he was older—it was pretty easy.

Potty training is a process. Once you start, keep that in mind. It's just not a one-and-done long-weekend kind of thing. Some kids might master peeing in the potty before pooping in the potty—that's normal. Nighttime training can take much, much longer than daytime training, sometimes years, with occasional accidents after that—and that's normal too. There really is very little you can do about nighttime dryness. Kids are not aware of peeing during their sleep, so short of waking them up, they will be dry when they are dry.

While you're potty training, keep the process positive. Try not to use negative adjectives like "gross" and "stinky" to describe going to the bathroom or pees and poops. Use plain language and call body parts and bodily waste by their proper names (I don't mean you have to say "bowel movement"—but you want to avoid calling poop something cutesy that obscures what's actually happening; the point is to normalize using the potty.) Help your child feel in charge of the process—toddlers want control. Talk to your child about how he or she gets to be in charge of his or her body now. When it comes to the specifics of how-to, there are countless potty-training books available, each with its own approach and philosophy. It can be overwhelming for parents to choose the right one. I suggest assessing whether a book's approach aligns with your parenting style and your child's temperament. Remember that each method is likely to insist its way is the only or best way. The truth is, there is no one-size-fits-all method, so it's essential to find an approach that feels comfortable and natural for both you and your child.

In terms of when to worry, urologists and doctors usually consider pee accidents a concern when an inability to toilet independently starts impeding a child's life, such as an inability to participate in sports, go to sleepovers, or attend sleepaway camp.

When it came to my patient Ethan, I wasn't worried at all and told his mom as much. I reassured Stephanie that every child is different and suggested she and her husband step back and follow Ethan's lead. Together, they decided to take a break from potty training for a few months and to enroll Ethan in a day care that didn't require children in the first year of the program to be potty trained. Next time I saw Ethan, I waited for him to come out of the bathroom to start his visit. He proudly announced he had gone on the potty. You get used to a lot of pee and poop talk as a pediatrician.

Elimination Communication

Over the last few years, quite a few parents have started asking me about elimination communication (EC), otherwise known as infant toilet training. At first, I was a little surprised (virtually no one asked me about it when I started practicing pediatrics). Since I run an integrative practice, it makes sense to me: EC is the norm in many Asian and African countries, which some of my natural-minded families tend to view as having more "traditional"—and therefore desirable—childcare practices. What is EC, if you're not one of those already familiar with it? Well, "infant toilet training" is your first clue. In EC, when babies (as young as newborns) need to pee or poop, a parent holds them bare-bottomed over a waste receptacle (often a toilet, but this could also just be a bucket). How do they know when their little potato is going to release a number one or number two? The answer to that is the heart of EC: they learn their child's cues. But there's a third piece to the puzzle—while the baby is going to the bathroom, the parent is supposed to make a sound specific to pottying (like "siss siss siss," for example). The idea is that the baby will learn to associate the sound with going pee or poop and that it will become a cue the parent can use to get the baby to go on command. End result: no (or fewer) diapers. Whether or not EC works, or works well, is a matter of debate that hinges on personal values and preferences. I'm not here to legislate how other cultures (or you) toilet train. In hearing from parents in my own practice who have attempted EC, the method doesn't train children to go to the toilet (i.e., to recognize their own body signals and hold their bladder or bowels), as much as it teaches parents to recognize their child's signals. If you want to try it, there's no reason not to go for it. But "should" you try it? No, I don't think you need to.

BODY EXPLORATION

Toddlers touch themselves. I like to be matter-of-fact about this topic to emphasize how *normal* it is. One of the ways children learn about themselves and the world around them during this time is by engaging in body exploration. Their curiosity about their bodies is a totally normal, age-appropriate, and essential part of their development. And typically you can expect it to include touching, examining, and even playing with their genitals. Trust me. It will happen. The most important thing you need to understand about this is: this behavior is *not* sexually motivated. It's a way for toddlers to understand their body and its sensations. And as with any behavior that causes a sensation that is interesting, new, or feels good, your toddler will likely repeat it—still not sexually. Your kid is not a deviant because he or she keeps putting a hand down the ol' diaper. (My own wife was concerned for a while that our son was a little too interested in his private parts—I reassured her many times it was normal. I'm still not sure she's convinced.)

Because toddlers are so curious about bodies and their differences, they might also be curious about seeing you naked or ask unfiltered questions about body parts. Many moms of boys can attest to the classic query, "Mama, why don't you have a penis?" Dads may get a vagina question or two. Dads, don't sweat it. You got this.

It's also totally normal for toddlers or preschoolers to touch/rub their genitals in public (not just in private—remember, this is like touching any other part of their body for them), try to look at or touch a peer's or sibling's genitals, show their genitals to peers, or try to see peers or adults naked. Of course, just because those behaviors are normal doesn't mean they are always safe or appropriate. As parents, our role is to help our kids learn about their bodies and healthy boundaries around them—without shame.

TODDLER PLAY

What is "play," and why does it matter? Before diving into practicalities, let's take a moment to explore the essence of play. It's not just a filler activity or a way to pass time; play is the work of childhood. It's a serious business for toddlers, filled with exploration, experimentation, and learning. According to research, play is crucial for a child's physical, emotional, and cognitive development. In today's consumer culture, it's easy to think that good parenting involves a lot of buying—more toys, more gadgets, more stuff. However, the most valuable gift you can give a child is your undivided attention during playtime. Expensive toys are not necessary. In fact, often the simplest items or even just your interactions can spur the most profound learning and joy. So many parents have purchased an expensive gift, only for the child to play with the box, the bubble cushioning, or the stickers that come with the toy.

Parents often feel pressured to "entertain" their kids, turning play into a performance. The aim of play isn't to dazzle your child with your storytelling prowess or arts and crafts skills; it's about engagement. It's an opportunity for you to come down to your child's level and see the world from his or her perspective. In this digital age, there's an overwhelming array of activities and games suggested online for every age group. It can be tempting to seek out novel ways to play, especially if you find play monotonous. Don't overlook the importance of repetition for toddlers. For them, doing the same thing over and over is a learning process, reinforcing cognitive and motor skills.

Imagination is a playground we should not forget about, and for a toddler, the whole world is an invitation to explore. Encourage play without toys: use household items, go out into nature, or simply engage in dialogue. Eli and I have gone on many a treasure hunt. We have a large pile of rocks and leaves outside our house.

It may surprise you, but play is a common discussion in my office. It was a sunny afternoon when Daniel walked in—his two-and-a-half-year-old daughter, Ling, in tow. He looked concerned but hopeful as he explained, "Doctor, Ling doesn't seem to play like the other kids her age.

She never plays alone, either. I am always having to come up with activities for us to do together. I wonder if there's anything we should be doing differently." After discussing diet, sleep, and general health, I suggested incorporating more unstructured play into her daily routine.

"Try this," I said, handing him a simple wooden puzzle and some colorful stacking blocks. "Let Ling explore these toys at her own pace. Don't guide her, just observe." We watched as she began to experiment, her eyes widened with curiosity, and she giggled with delight. Daniel looked amazed. I shared, "You see, play is not just 'free time' or a break from learning. It *is* learning. Through play, Ling will learn to problem-solve, fine-tune motor skills, and even pick up social cues." A few weeks later, they returned, his face glowing with a newfound optimism. Ling had transformed into a bubbly, more energetic child, and it was clear that the power of play had worked its magic, and she was often playing on her own.

It's beneficial for your child to sometimes take the lead during playtime. It allows him or her to feel empowered and fosters creativity. By merely following your child's lead, you allow your child to take charge of his or her own learning experience. It's not all about playing together, though. Encouraging independent play is not neglectful; it's nurturing a vital skill. Independent play fosters creativity, problem solving, and self-reliance. Research suggests that it can enhance emotional regulation and promote executive functions like planning and organizing. Parents often wonder when it's okay for a child to play independently. The truth is, even a two-year-old should be able to engage in short bursts of independent play. Setting up an environment conducive for self-play, like a Montessori shelf or accessible art supplies, can facilitate this process.

While it's essential to spend time playing with your child, the quality of the interaction is more critical than the duration. You don't need to spend seven hours a day in dedicated play. Moments of intense connection, where you are entirely present for your child, can be more meaningful than a full day of distracted, half-hearted play. In conclusion, play is a versatile and vital tool in your parenting toolbox. It's a means of connection, a facilitator of growth, and a foundation for a lifetime of learning. Remember that your presence and engagement are the most crucial elements in enriching your child's world through play.

As we close this section, let's remember that the essence of parenting lies in tuning in to your child's unique pace and needs. Navigating this transition can be both exhilarating and challenging, but the key is to approach it with a sense of wonder, openness, and adaptability. Just as your child is growing and learning, so are you. The shift from baby to toddler is not just a developmental leap for your child, but also a transformative experience for you as a parent. So take a deep breath, trust yourself and your child, and embrace the extraordinary journey ahead.

Health and Wellness

GETTING SICK

As children begin to interact more with the world around them, especially when they go to day care or preschool, their immune systems are frequently tested. I warn every parent who is sending a child to school for the first time to be ready for the inevitable revolving door of colds that are coming the family's way. Understanding some of the common illnesses kids may contract can help caregivers detect, manage, and sometimes prevent them.

PREVENTION AND IMMUNE SUPPORT

While illnesses are a common part of early childhood, there are steps to bolster immunity and reduce risk. Teach your children proper handwashing and practice good hygiene at home. Focus on the SEEDS of well-being—stress, environment, exercise (activity), diet, and sleep. And don't forget about the Dr. Gator smoothie!

As a quick reminder, always consult your pediatrician or health-care provider when you're concerned about your child's health or if symptoms seem severe. Early intervention can sometimes prevent complications.

Most common childhood illnesses are caused by either bacterial or viral infections. Both bacteria and viruses are types of microorganisms, but they are fundamentally different when it comes to their structure, how they reproduce, and how we treat them medically. Bacteria are single-celled organisms with a simple cellular structure that includes a cell membrane, cytoplasm, and DNA. They can live independently, reproduce by dividing in half, and can be beneficial or harmful. Antibiotics can often treat bacterial infections. In contrast, viruses are much smaller and are not cellular; instead, they consist of genetic material (DNA or RNA) encased in a protein coat. Viruses cannot live or reproduce on their own; they must infect a host cell to carry out their life cycle. Antiviral medications, *not* antibiotics, are required to treat viral infections. The bad news is that antivirals do not exist for most viruses. The good news is that most viruses don't require treatment with medication.

Here's an important distinction to remember: while a child who contracts a bacterial infection will usually require medication, a child who contracts a viral infection will likely not. The majority of childhood illness is caused by viruses and the vast, vast, vast majority of the time, your child does not need a medication to heal. Antibiotics don't treat viruses.

Common Early Childhood and Toddler Illnesses

Colds and Upper Respiratory Viral Infections—Caused by numerous viruses, colds are characterized by runny nose, cough, mild fever, and general discomfort.
Management: Rest, hydration, and saline drops for nasal congestion. Over-the-counter pain relievers can be used as directed for discomfort and fever.

Gastroenteritis (Stomach Bug)—A virus that manifests as vomiting, diarrhea, abdominal pain, and sometimes fever. It can lead to dehydration.
Management: Focus on keeping your child hydrated with small sips of oral rehydration solutions. If dehydration signs appear or symptoms persist, seek medical care.

Otitis Media (Middle Ear Infection)—Common symptoms include ear pain, fever, irritability, and sometimes fluid discharge.
Management: Consult your pediatrician. You may be able to watchfully wait and manage pain. The doctor may prescribe antibiotics if the infection is prolonged or considered bacterial. Pain can be managed with over-the-counter pain relievers.

Croup—A viral illness identifiable by a distinctive "barking" cough and sometimes difficulty breathing.
Management: Keep your child calm, as crying can exacerbate symptoms. Cool night air or a steamy bathroom can help. Seek medical care if breathing difficulties increase.

Hand, Foot, and Mouth Disease—A viral illness with symptoms like fever, sore throat, and painful blisters on the hands, feet, and inside the mouth.
Management: Symptomatic treatment with pain relievers and cold foods. It typically resolves within a week.

Bronchiolitis—A respiratory infection affecting tiny airways in the lungs, often caused by respiratory syncytial virus (RSV). Symptoms include wheezing, difficulty breathing, and cough.
Management: Ensure hydration and consult a pediatrician.

Roseola—A viral illness characterized by a sudden high fever followed by a rosy-pink rash.
Management: Use fever-reducing medications as needed. Once the rash appears, the illness typically soon resolves.

Thrush (Oral Candidiasis)—A fungal infection resulting in white patches inside the mouth and on the tongue, which can be painful.
Management: Consult your pediatrician, who may prescribe an antifungal medication.

Fifth Disease (Erythema Infectiosum)—Also caused by a virus, it presents as a "slapped cheek" red rash on the face and can spread to the body.
Management: It's usually mild and resolves on its own. Pain relievers can help manage symptoms.

PRESCRIPTION AND OTC MEDICATION FOR BABIES AND TODDLERS

Navigating the world of pediatric medication can be daunting. With so many options available, it's often challenging to determine the best course of action, especially when our children are in distress. As an integrative-minded pediatrician, I have spent years considering how and when to use traditional medicines versus natural remedies, with a child's well-being always my primary goal. In today's fast-paced world, there's an increasing trend to seek quick fixes. As a result, many children are often given medication as a first line of treatment, even when less invasive measures might suffice. Overmedication can lead to potential side effects, drug interactions, and even bacteria that are resistant to antibiotics.

Little Shandy, a three-year-old with moderate right ear pain, was taken to urgent care by her worried parents. Without an in-depth examination, Shandy was promptly prescribed antibiotics. This is a common narrative in medical facilities. Confused, her parents called me to see if she really needed the medication. She did not have a fever and, after the drive home, already seemed to be feeling better and was back to her usual self. The fact is, not all ear infections require antibiotics. Often the cause of ear pain is viral and the symptoms will resolve on their own, or they have noninfectious causes like teething. According to the AAP, you can often wait to treat ear pain with antibiotics for forty-eight hours unless there are high fevers or extreme pain.

The reality is that medications and especially antibiotics are overprescribed. Sometimes an antibiotic can save your life, so, of course, I am extremely thankful antibiotics exist. That does not mean you should haphazardly pop antibiotics like candy at the mere sign of a sniffle or the first indication of ear pain. It is important to note again that most infections and illnesses are viruses. As mentioned earlier, viruses are not treated by antibiotics. There are few greater examples of this than in the evaluation of ear pain. This is not woo-woo, alternative medicine. Antibiotic stewardship is important. Antibiotics kill bad bacteria, but they also kill *good* bacteria. Only give antibiotics to your kids when they *truly* need them.

In my experience, there are a few medications that natural-minded parents and not so natural-minded parents alike will keep in their bathroom cabinet, "just in case," such as Tylenol (acetaminophen), Motrin (ibuprofen) and Benadryl (diphenhydramine). (Though there are brands of these drugs with better ingredients that parents are starting to turn to more frequently, such as Genexa.) Over-the-counter medications for children usually come up in the context of fever (which we dig into in the next section). As we will discuss, there is certainly something to be said for letting a fever run its course. Generally, if your child has a fever, you should be in contact with your pediatrician to discuss best steps and decide if a visit is needed. When it is indicated to use acetaminophen or ibuprofen to reduce fever, there is some evidence that alternating fever medication therapy may be more effective at reducing temperatures than monotherapy alone. With both acetaminophen and ibuprofen, it's important to adhere to recommended dosages to avoid potential side effects. Antihistamines are another common over-the-counter medication that a pediatrician may recommend to treat allergies and hives. Some can cause drowsiness, so always follow age-specific recommendations.

WHEN TO WORRY ABOUT BABIES AND TODDLERS

As your child gets older, it is often much easier to decide when to be worried. Certainly, once your child can talk, he or she can let you know he or she stepped on something sharp or ate some dog poop at the park (yep, that's happened). The more you get to know your child, the easier it will be to know when to be worried. Your frame of reference evolves over time. This is the likely reason parents of first children call me when the wind blows the wrong way, yet parents of third children don't call me at all unless their kid's arm is falling off.

Let's get into some specifics:

Fever—there is a lot of fever phobia. Maybe we over-scare you in the newborn period without properly explaining fever. In the first month or two, if a newborn gets a fever, he or she can get sick very quickly, so doctors treat a newborn fever differently than they would after two months. In general, fever is actually a good thing. It is part of your body's natural defense against disease. We raise our temperature to make the body a less habitable place for the infection. When your child gets sick, he or she will often have a fever. A normal cold/virus lasts about three to five days. Fevers can bounce around for a few days. Normal fevers for a virus run about 100–103 degrees. Sometimes fevers can even run 103–105. If your child consistently has fevers above 103, you should get him or her evaluated. Higher temperatures more likely connote a bacterial disease, but they can still be caused by regular old colds. If your child has fevers for more than five days, he or she should always be seen. Usually, children should get checked after two to three days of fever. We aren't necessarily worried at that point, but it is worth a look.

So, when do we worry about fevers or children in general? Usually, it is the symptoms *that accompany* a fever—like fever coupled with extreme pain, fever combined with trouble breathing, and fever with lethargy—that are cause for concern. What do doctors worry about? Here is a quick list of some of the biggies.

- Extreme pain: With a baby, crying is our main indicator of pain, but it can be hard to localize and needs some detective work. If an older child says the lower right part of their belly hurts, you can put away your magnifying glass, Sherlock. Increasing and severe pain is always a concern and should be evaluated.

- Breathing: Any breathing concerns always need to be seen. Is your child coughing, wheezing, turning blue? These will all need a visit STAT.

- Pre-existing condition with new symptoms: Does your child have another medical condition like diabetes, autism, lupus? We are generally more concerned about any child with other conditions as he or she is more likely to get sicker, faster.

- Lethargy/acting abnormal: Has there been an acute change in mental status? Is your child not waking up? Is he or she unable to get off the couch? Is your child acting funny, talking funny? This needs to be seen ASAP.

- Trauma: "Do you think it could be broken, doc?" While I am pretty good, I don't quite have X-ray vision yet. Luckily, we do have machines that do. If you feel the injury was bad enough that a bone could be broken, it is usually best to get evaluated.

A WELLNESS "MEDICINE" CHEST FOR BABIES AND TODDLERS: NATURAL REMEDIES AND SUPPLEMENTS

In my office, I emphasize the importance of an integrative approach to pediatric health. While traditional medicines are invaluable, understanding their proper use and supplementing them with natural remedies can offer a holistic approach to children's well-being. It's always essential to consult with a health-care professional before making any medical decisions for your child.

As with newborns, I still think vitamin D, omegas, and probiotics have a place in your baby and toddler's wellness arsenal. For more information on these three supplements, please revisit "A Wellness 'Medicine' Chest for Newborns" (p. 115) for more details. Other remedies and supplements to consider as children get older include:

Vitamin C: This antioxidant can aid in tissue repair and improve immune function.

Zinc: Plays a vital role in immune function. Deficiency can lead to an increased susceptibility to infections.

Multivitamins: Ensure children get all essential vitamins and minerals, especially if they are picky eaters.

Elderberry: Often used as a natural support for colds and flu due to its antiviral properties, elderberry is one of my go-to immune support supplements. That's why I created my very own organic elderberry syrup through my Tiny Roots Apothecary supplement line. Elderberry refers to several different varieties of the *Sambucus* tree, which is a flowering plant belonging to the Adoxaceae family. The most common type is *Sambucus nigra,* also known as the European elderberry or black elder. This tree is native to Europe, though it is widely grown in many other parts of the world as well. What makes elderberry a good resource for wellness support? Elderberry is:

- High in vitamin C
- High in dietary fiber

- A good source of phenolic acids. These compounds are potent antioxidants that can help reduce damage from oxidative stress in the body.

- A good source of flavonols. Elderberry contains the antioxidant flavonols quercetin, kaempferol, and isorhamnetin.

- Rich in anthocyanins. These compounds give the fruit its characteristic dark black-purple color and are a strong antioxidant with anti-inflammatory effects.

I'm genuinely surprised elderberry is still viewed as woo-woo by so many in modern medicine. Numerous published studies on the benefits of elderberry exist, and minimal risk has been found. Nothing is without risk, but to me, the risks from a berry/supplement are almost always a lot lower than medications. In my opinion, the scientific literature says, YES, it can be helpful in respiratory viral illness. Manufacturers can't make medical claims about a supplement in the US, so I can't tell you what to do, but I do recommend elderberry for bronchial support to my patients and use it myself. The research is not perfect; it depends on which study you review. The effects of elderberry are not extreme, but then again, you should not expect extreme effects from a berry.

The Nontoxic Home

Home: for many of us it represents safety—it's a sanctuary, a refuge, a place of comfort and warmth. Keeping our homes clean—not to mention decorating and furnishing them, *especially* a nursery—is a way of caring not only for our living space, but for our well-being. Unfortunately, many of the products that promise to make our homes cozy and sparkling are, with ongoing exposure, harmful to our health. From cleaning products to laundry detergent, from clothing to bedding, from air fresheners and candles to furniture, many common household items contain known endocrine disruptors, air pollutants, and respiratory and skin irritants. Kiddos, with their rapidly developing bodies and immature immune systems, are even more susceptible to these environmental invaders than adults (especially since they spend a lot of time playing on the floor, touch everything, and have a habit of putting their hands—and toys—in their mouth).

Some of the main culprits to look out for when it comes to environmental toxins include:

- **Volatile Organic Compounds, aka VOCs:** VOCs are chemicals that vaporize at room temperature—meaning we then inhale them. VOCs can cause, contribute to, and exacerbate chronic respiratory disease and illness (such as asthma), among other health concerns. Common VOCs include formaldehyde, ammonia, bleach, and benzene. Common sources of VOCs include household cleaning products (like glass and oven cleaners), air fresheners (yes, even the fancy ones), scented candles, dry-cleaning chemicals, furniture (especially furniture made of pressed wood, pressboard, and medium-density fiberboard), and paint.
- **Phthalates, aka "The Everywhere Chemical":** Phthalates are man-made chemical compounds invented in the last century to help make plastics more flexible. Today, they're used as stabilizers in countless cosmetic and personal care products, particularly in products that contain fragrance. Personal care products that may contain phthalates include lotions, bodywash, shampoo, conditioner, nail polish, hair

spray, and perfume, among others. Household products that may include phthalates include air fresheners, scented cleaning products, and all plastics. Phthalates have been shown to be endocrine disruptors, which have negative long-term impacts on child growth and development, the reproductive systems in both young children and adolescents, pregnancy, and fertility.

- **Perfluorochemicals, aka PFCs, and Per- and Poly-Fluoroalkyl Substances, aka PFAs or "Forever Chemicals":** PFCs and PFAs are another group of man-made chemicals that are used in many products to make coatings that resist heat, oil, stains, grease, and water. PFCs and PFAs are commonly found in nonstick cookware, clothing (like rain jackets), furniture, rugs, and even food packaging. PFCs and PFAs are not naturally found in the environment, but they persist in it for a very long time, building up in wildlife and our waterways. PFCs have been linked to inflammation, disrupted endocrine function, immune system dysfunction, and respiratory disease.

- **Flame Retardants:** Flame retardants are a class of chemical compositions that are applied to flammable materials to prevent burning or slow the spread of fire—there are hundreds of different flame retardants. Among the most concerning are brominated flame retardants, which can build up in tissue and have been linked to cancer and endocrine disruption, and in 2020 were found to be an even greater concern than lead when it comes to environmental contributors to intellectual disability in children. Flame retardants are commonly used in mattresses, textiles (bedding, pajamas, furniture upholstery), nursing pillows, strollers, and car seats.

I know that for parents and caregivers (heck, for anyone who cares about their long-term health), learning that there are so many harmful toxins lurking in our everyday environment can be overwhelming. Our desire to protect our children is both innate and incredibly powerful, so the realization that potential harm lies in everyday household items can feel daunting when it comes to where to start to better safeguard our families from their effects. My best advice to combat the overwhelm has two simple components: focus on air quality and focus on the products you use the most.

When it comes to home air quality, control dust—vacuum regularly, using a vacuum with a HEPA filter if you can. Dust can contain lead, PFAs, flame retardants, phthalates, etc., shed by our walls, furniture, and carpeting. Add as many air-cleaning plants like aloe or spider plants as is feasible (and that you won't kill, lol). Open your windows! Ventilation is important to bring fresh air into the home; people are surprised to learn that indoor air quality is often worse than outdoor air quality.

When it comes to focusing on the products you use the most, instead of setting out on a huge Marie Kondo–esque journey to go through every single product or object in your household, start by switching out the things you use daily, especially body care, and that you sleep in or on. For everything else, replace as you go; read labels and look for products that are phthalate- and PFC-free, have low or no VOCs, and are made of organic materials and ingredients. Avoid plastics and synthetic fragrance in general. If you're just getting started on buying baby products, use the above information and the following suggestions for child-friendly choices as a beginner's guide.

Child-Friendly Choices for a Nontoxic Home

Cleaning Products

- Vinegar and water mix as an all-purpose cleaner
- Baking soda for scouring tasks

Air Fresheners and Scented Products

- Diffusers with child-safe essential oils
- Use child-safe essential oils to scent homemade cleaners
- Candles that are 100 percent beeswax-, soy-, or coconut-based; unscented candles or candles that are scented only with essential oils; candles that have 100 percent cotton, hemp, or wood wicks

Bedding and Clothing

- Mattresses and pillows made of organic cotton, wool, coconut coir, or natural latex made from rubber trees and free of polyurethane foam and flame retardants

- Tight-fitting pajamas made of 100 percent organic cotton or bamboo free of flame retardants; wool sleep sacks free of flame retardants
- 100 percent organic cotton, bamboo, or wool blankets and sheets free of flame retardants

Furniture, Household Items and Baby Gear

- Solid wood furniture and toys without chemical finishes
- Furniture certified to be low in VOCs (volatile organic compounds)
- Stainless steel, ceramic, and cast-iron cookware
- Car seats and strollers that are flame retardant- and PFC-free
- Natural and organic rubber, fabric, and wood toys

Finally, I wouldn't be a truly natural-minded, integrative pediatrician if I didn't address the ever-increasing barrage of wireless "smart" devices in our homes that rely on Bluetooth and Wi-Fi connections and the omnipresence of cellular and computing devices in our lives, all of which create electric and magnetic fields (EMFs), which are invisible areas of energy. Though the type of "nonionizing" EMFs produced by our devices are generally considered to contain only low-level radiation that is not regarded as dangerous to humans, there is ongoing research dedicated to studying the effects of EMFs, given our increasing exposure to them. Some studies have already suggested a link between EMF exposure and potential health risks, especially among children, including disturbances in sleep patterns, potential behavioral changes, and changes at the cellular level. In my opinion, given this is a new field of study and that cellular signals become more powerful each year, it is prudent to be mindful of the way EMFs may affect our children long-term and take basic and common-sense precautions to minimize risk, including:

- Keeping Wi-Fi routers away from children's bedrooms, and turning them off at night
- Using wired connections when possible
- Educating children about limiting screen time and keeping devices at a safe distance from their bodies.

Creating a nontoxic home for children isn't just about shielding them from immediate harm; it's about fostering a healthy environment where they can thrive without unnecessary exposure to environmental toxins and hazards that may create *long-term* harm. By being mindful of our small, everyday choices, we can make significant strides toward ensuring our homes are safe havens for our little ones.

Conclusion

From the moment you learn you're going to become a parent, your life undergoes a tectonic shift. This transition isn't just about additional responsibilities or adding a new member to your household; it's about an alteration of your very identity, priorities, and perspective. Everything you once knew, from your daily routines to your aspirations, starts to orbit around the new life you've brought into the world. As with any significant change, challenges are inevitable. Yet, with each challenge comes an unparalleled joy and depth of experience.

Embracing this shift doesn't mean leaving behind who you were, but expanding your identity to encompass the nurturing, protective, and ever-adapting role of a parent. Exemplary parenting stems from a well-nourished self. It's from the reservoir of personal wellness that we draw patience, kindness, calm, and resilience. Parenthood, while infinitely rewarding, is undeniably demanding. The days of uninterrupted sleep and leisurely evenings feel like relics of a bygone era. Amid the cacophony of diaper changes, day care runs, and endless rounds of peek-a-boo, it becomes paramount for parents to find pockets of serenity. These moments of calm aren't just luxuries; they're essential for mental, emotional, and physical well-being. It might be a few stolen moments with a book, a quiet evening walk, or a cherished hobby. Amid the delightful whirlwind that is parenting, discovering and holding on to these peaceful moments ensures that you remain grounded and rejuvenated.

Parenting is a profound journey rather than a fixed destination. It is continuously shaped and enriched by the experiences we share, the knowledge we acquire, and the unwavering love we give and receive. Embrace a holistic approach by striving to be whole, present, and nurturing. One of the most effective ways to enrich this journey is by learning to manage personal stress. While stress might feel like an overwhelming force, it is essentially a biological mechanism meant to prompt us to reassess, adapt, and evolve. As parents, it's crucial to recognize and respond to these signals appropriately.

In today's fast-paced world, the pressure to keep up with the parental status quo is immense. Of course, we all want to ensure that our children have everything they need while safeguarding them from life's numerous challenges. However, it's important to remember that there is no need to constantly measure your family against others. Every child and every family has its own unique rhythm, and recognizing this helps you to parent at a pace that's appropriate for your family's individual needs. I encourage you to feel confident in making decisions that are right for *your* family, always within the parameters of what is considered safe by scientific literature. Trust in your innate parental intuition—your "mama or papa gut"—which plays a crucial role in this process.

Being well-informed about the scientific research surrounding parenting practices is undeniably important, as it provides a basis for well-considered decisions that are in consensus with the latest findings. Nevertheless, it's equally important to acknowledge that there are few absolutes in parenting. The field is so diverse and dynamic that there is seldom only one correct approach for all situations. You know your family better than anyone else—better than your own parents, your doctor, or your inquisitive neighbor. You are the lifeblood of your family unit, and ultimately, you will make the decisions that best support and nurture your loved ones. There may be occasions when those decisions diverge from mainstream thought, but what matters most is that they're made with love, care, and an informed perspective. In an era saturated with prescriptive parenting manuals, social media portrayals of flawless family life, and daunting yardsticks of "success," it is essential to tune out the clamor, set aside the digital distractions, and adopt a concept of "good enough" parenting that unfolds at your child's natural pace.

Chasing the mirage of perfection not only drains the delight from parenting but also imposes on you unattainable standards that benefit no one. The truth is, perfect parenting is a myth. Each day, we strive to do our best, we learn, we evolve, and we press on. Parenting is an evolutionary process, reflective of the undulating path of life itself. It's the cumulative effect of daily incremental steps, mindful choices, and a dedicated commitment to nurturing your child's holistic growth that truly counts over time.

The parent who is engaged and attentive will invariably outshine the one who believes that material possessions or a meticulously curated social media presence can pave the way to a well-adjusted child. It's not the accumulation of things that defines parenting prowess. The odds are your child will not hold on to the memory of the toy he or she received at age two. Your child *will* cherish and remember the times spent with a parent who was truly there with him or her—engaged and participating in the moment.

Here's a little perspective to leave you with: In America, the average amount of time moms spend with their children is **120 minutes a day**. The average amount of time dads spend with their children is just **85 minutes a day**. About **75 percent** of the time we spend with our kids in our lifetime happens **before they are twelve years old**. We have about eighteen summers with our kids. Remember to slow down and BE PRESENT. Enjoy your precious little time with them because it will soon be over. While the milestones of life—birthdays, first steps, and first words—are undeniably special, it's often the everyday moments that linger in our and our children's memories. A spontaneous picnic, bedtime stories that turn into prolonged discussions about the universe, or even shared household chores can become the threads that weave the fabric of your family's unique narrative. It's not about grand gestures. It *is* about listening and sharing experiences. These shared moments, both profound and mundane, form the indelible memories that define your family's journey.

Trust in your ability to be the perfect parent for YOUR FAMILY. Embrace the journey, relish in the love, and remember, you are doing a fantastic job. And in the grand scheme, isn't this love and connection the real magic smoothie we have been seeking all along? Let's raise our proverbial smoothie glasses to this incredible journey called parenting—one filled with challenges, triumphs, lessons, and, most important, resilience. Your child's health and well-being start with *you*—calm, confident, and caring. Stay strong, keep learning, and continue to care deeply. In doing so, you are not just building a healthier child, but a healthier world as well. Cheers to you, dear parent!

You've got this.

Recommended Resources

General Health and Guidelines

- **CDC:** Comprehensive information on children's health, vaccines, developmental milestones, and more.
  www.cdc.gov

- **AAP:** Evidence-based guidelines and recommendations on pediatric care.
  www.aap.org

Research Databases

- **PubMed:** Deep dive into scientific literature related to pediatric health.
  pubmed.ncbi.nlm.nih.gov

Newborn Care

- **Newborn Weight:** A tool to track your newborn's weight and guidelines for early weeks.
  newbornweight.org/

Car Safety

- **NHTSA:** Guidelines and recommendations about car seats and booster seats.
  www.nhtsa.gov/equipment/car-seats-and-booster-seats

Breastfeeding Support

- **Women's Health:** Comprehensive information and support for breastfeeding mothers.
  www.womenshealth.gov/breastfeeding

- **Medela:** Educational materials and products to assist with breastfeeding.
  www.medela.us/breastfeeding/breastfeeding-support/breastfeeding-university
- **Lactation Network:** Connecting you to lactation consultants and offering breastfeeding support.
  lactationnetwork.com
- **NCBI Bookshelf LactMed:** A digital library of life sciences and health-care publications on lactation medications/supplements.
  www.ncbi.nlm.nih.gov/books/NBK501922/

Food and Nutrition

- **FDA CFR:** Code of Federal Regulations for infant formula.
  www.accessdata.fda.gov/scripts/cdrh/cfdocs/cfcfr/CFRSearch.cfm?fr=107.100

First Aid

- **Red Cross:** Online courses in child and baby first aid, CPR, and Automated External Defibrillator (AED).
  www.redcross.org/take-a-class/classes/child-and-baby-first-aid%2Fcpr%2Faed-online-ol/a6R3o000001vv2U.html

Parenting and Well-Being

- **Healthy Children:** Parent-friendly articles and tips from the AAP.
  www.healthychildren.org/
- **Global Health Media:** Informational content on global health issues for children.
  globalhealthmedia.org

- **CDC Growth and Milestones:** Standard growth charts and milestone information.

  Growth Charts:
  www.cdc.gov/growthcharts

  Milestones:
  www.cdc.gov/ncbddd/actearly/milestones/index.html

  ***Milestone Moments* booklet:**
  www.cdc.gov/ncbddd/actearly/pdf/parents_pdfs/
  milestonemomentseng508.pdf

Language Development

- **American Speech-Language-Hearing Association:** Guide for understanding speech and language developmental milestones.
  www.asha.org/public/speech/development/

Toddler

- **Siggie Cohen website:** Includes fantastic resources and courses for normal toddler behavior.
  drsiggie.com

- **Tina Payne Bryson Website and Books:** A wealth of information on pediatric mental health. Popular books include *The Whole-Brain Child* and *No-Drama Discipline*.
  www.tinabryson.com

- **Emily Oster ParentData and book *Cribsheets*:** A data driven analysis on parenting.
  parentdata.org/

- **Janet Lansbury:** *No Bad Kids* (book and courses).
  www.janetlansbury.com/

Environmental Protection

- **US Environmental Protection Agency:**
  Safe Drinking Water Information Hotline: 1-800-426-4791;
  Emergency Response Hotline: 1-800-424-8802.

Starting Solids

- **Solid Starts:** A resource for introducing solid foods to infants.
  solidstarts.com/

Healthy Foods

- **EWG:** A list of foods to consider for their nutritional value and safety.
  www.ewg.org/foodnews/full-list.php

Integrative Health

- **Raising Amazing Plus:** Dr. Gator's website with a variety of courses on holistic health.
  www.raisingamazingplus.com

References

SECTION I: ARRIVAL

"About Baby Friendly USA." Baby Friendly USA. www.babyfriendlyusa.org /about/.

The American College of Obstetrics and Gynecologists. "Delayed Umbilical Cord Clamping After Birth." www.acog.org/clinical/clinical-guidance/committee -opinion/articles/2020/12/delayed-umbilical-cord-clamping-after-birth.

Andersson, Ola, Barbro Lindquist, Magnus Lindgren, Karin Stjernqvist, Magnus Domellöf, and Lena Hellström-Westas. "Effect of Delayed Cord Clamping on Neurodevelopment at 4 Years of Age: A Randomized Clinical Trial." *JAMA Pediatrics* 169 (2015): 631–638. doi.org/10.1001/jamapediatrics.2015.0358.

Barrera, Chloe M., Jennifer M. Nelson, Ellen O. Boundy, and Cria G. Perrine. "Trends in Rooming-In Practices Among Hospitals in the United States, 2007–2015." *Birth* 45, no. 4 (December 2018): 432–439.

Be The Match. "How Does a Patient's Ethnic Background Affect Matching?" bethematch.org/transplant-basics/how-marrow-transplants-work/how-does-a -patients-ethnic-background-affect-matching/.

Bossio, Jennifer A., Caroline F. Pukall, and Stephen S. Steele. "Examining Penile Sensitivity in Neonatally Circumcised and Intact Men Using Quantitative Sensory Testing." *Journal of Urology* 195, no. 6 (June 2016): 1848–1853.

Byakika-Tusiime, Jayne. "Circumcision and HIV Infection: Assessment of Causality." *AIDS Behavior* 12, no. 6 (November 2008): 835–841. doi.org/10.1007 /s10461-008-9453-6.

Cancer.org. "Penile Cancer Prevention." www.cancer.org/cancer/penile-cancer /causes-risks-prevention/prevention.html.

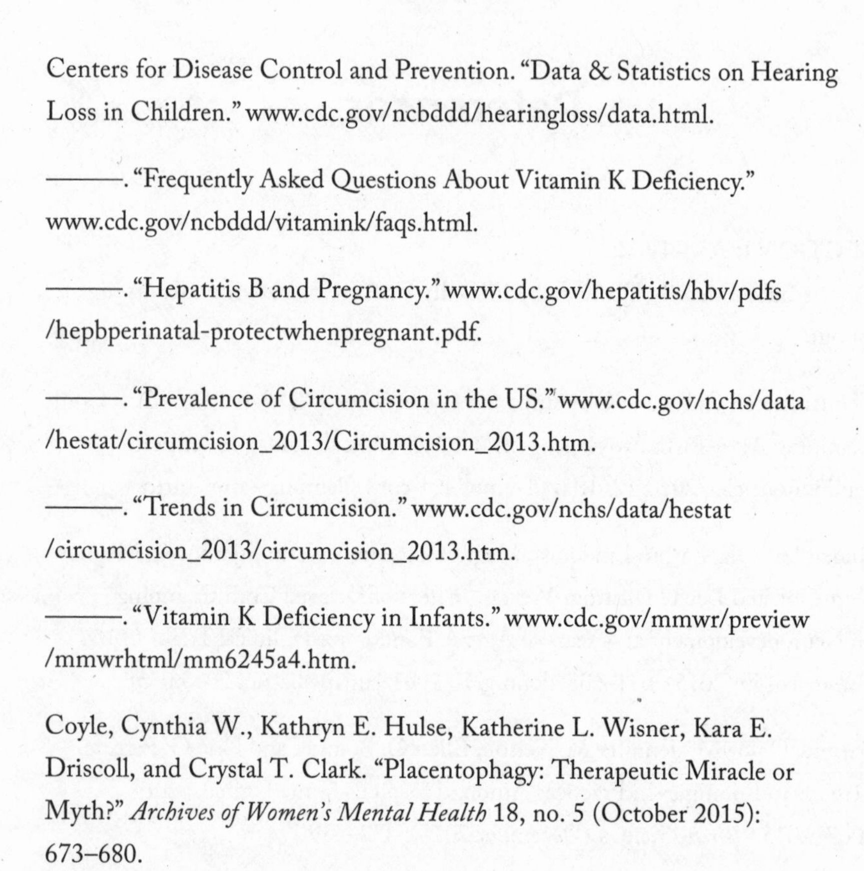

Centers for Disease Control and Prevention. "Data & Statistics on Hearing Loss in Children." www.cdc.gov/ncbddd/hearingloss/data.html.

———. "Frequently Asked Questions About Vitamin K Deficiency." www.cdc.gov/ncbddd/vitamink/faqs.html.

———. "Hepatitis B and Pregnancy." www.cdc.gov/hepatitis/hbv/pdfs/hepbperinatal-protectwhenpregnant.pdf.

———. "Prevalence of Circumcision in the US." www.cdc.gov/nchs/data/hestat/circumcision_2013/Circumcision_2013.htm.

———. "Trends in Circumcision." www.cdc.gov/nchs/data/hestat/circumcision_2013/circumcision_2013.htm.

———. "Vitamin K Deficiency in Infants." www.cdc.gov/mmwr/preview/mmwrhtml/mm6245a4.htm.

Coyle, Cynthia W., Kathryn E. Hulse, Katherine L. Wisner, Kara E. Driscoll, and Crystal T. Clark. "Placentophagy: Therapeutic Miracle or Myth?" *Archives of Women's Mental Health* 18, no. 5 (October 2015): 673–680.

The Cut. "What Is the Human Placenta Project?" 2019. www.thecut.com/2019/08/what-is-the-human-placenta-project.html.

Daling, Janet R., Margaret M. Madeleine, Lisa G. Johnson, Stephen M. Schwartz, Katherine A. Shera, Michelle A. Wurscher, Joseph J. Carter, Peggy L. Porter, Denise A. Galloway, James K. McDougall, and John N. Krieger. "Penile Cancer: Importance of Circumcision, Human Papillomavirus and Smoking in *In Situ* and Invasive Disease." *International Journal of Cancer* 116, no. 4 (2005): 606–616. doi.org/10.1002/ijc.21009.

Evidence Based Birth. "The Evidence for Skin-to-Skin Care After a Cesarean." evidencebasedbirth.com/the-evidence-for-skin-to-skin-care-after-a-cesarean/.

Hung, Ya-Ching, David C. Chang, Maggie L. Westfal, Isobel H. Marks, Peter T. Masiakos, and Cassandra M. Kelleher. "A Longitudinal Population Analysis of Cumulative Risks of Circumcision." *Journal of Surgical Research* 233 (2019): 111–117. doi.org/10.1016/j.jss.2018.07.069.

Introcaso, Camille E., Fujie Xu, Peter H. Kilmarx, Akbar Zaidi, and Lauri E. Markowitz. "Prevalence of Circumcision Among Men and Boys Aged 14 to 59 Years in the United States, National Health and Nutrition Examination Surveys 2005–2010." *Sexually Transmitted Diseases* 40, no. 7 (2013): 521–525.

Kuczmarski, Robert J., Cynthia L. Ogden, Shumei S. Guo, Laurence M. Grummer-Strawn, Katherine M. Flegal, Zuguo Mei, Rong Wei, Lester R. Curtin, Alex F. Roche, and Clifford L. Johnson. "2000 CDC Growth Charts for the United States: Methods and Development." *Vital Health Statistics* 11, no. 246 (2002): 1–190.

Lehmann, Jörgen. "Vitamin K as a Prophylactic in 13,000 Infants." CAB Direct. *The Lancet* 243, no. 6294 (1944): 493–494.

Levy, Tali, and Isaac Blickstein. "Timing of Cord Clamping Revisited." *Journal of Perinatal Medicine* 34 (2006): 293–297.

Linderkamp, Otwin. "Blood Rheology in the Newborn Infant." *Baillieres Clinical Haematology* l, no. 1 (1987): 801–825.

Linderkamp, Otwin, Mathias Nelle, Martina Kraus, and Eugen P. Zilow. "The Effect of Early and Late Cord-Clamping on Blood Viscosity and Other Hemorheological Parameters in Full-Term Neonates." *Acta Paediatrica* 81 (1992): 745–750.

Londish, Gregory J., and John M. Murray. "Significant Reduction in HIV Prevalence According to Male Circumcision Intervention in Sub-Saharan Africa." *International Journal of Epidemiology* 37, no. 6 (December 2008): 1246–1253. doi.org/10.1093/ije/dyn038.

Masood, S., H. R. H. Patel, R. C. Himpson, J. H. Palmer, G. R. Mufti, and M. K. M. Sheriff. "Penile Sensitivity and Sexual Satisfaction After Circumcision: Are We Informing Men Correctly?" *International Journal of Urology* 75, no. 1 (2005): 62–66. doi.org/10.1159/000085930.

Morris, Brian J., and John N. Krieger. "The Contrasting Evidence Concerning the Effect of Male Circumcision on Sexual Function, Sensation, and Pleasure: Systematic Review." *Sexual Medicine* 8, no. 4 (December 2020): 577–598.

Mota-Rojas, Daniel, Agustín Orihuela, Ana Strappini, Dina Villanueva-García, Fabio Napolitano, Patricia Mora-Medina, Hugo B. Barrios-García, Yuridia Herrera, Eunice Lavalle, and Julio Martínez-Burnes. "Consumption of Maternal Placenta in Humans and Nonhuman Mammals: Beneficial and Adverse Effects." *Animals (Basel)* 10, no. 12 (December 2020): 2398.

National Institute of Child Health and Human Development. "Newborn Screening Conditions." www.nichd.nih.gov/health/topics/newborn /conditioninfo/infants-screened.

———. "Podcast on Placenta Consumption." 2015. www.nichd.nih.gov /newsroom/releases/062615-podcast-placenta-consumption.

Ober, William B. "PLACENTOPHAGY." *Obstetrics & Gynecology* 41, no. 2 (February 1973): 317–318. journals.lww.com/greenjournal/Citation /1973/02000/PLACENTOPHAGY.32.aspx.

Oster, Emily. *Cribsheet*. New York: Penguin Press, 2019, pp. 16–17.

PDQ Adult Treatment Editorial Board. "Penile Cancer Treatment (PDQ®): Health Professional Version." June 2, 2023.

Pisacane, Alfredo. "Neonatal Prevention of Iron Deficiency." *BMJ* 312 (1996): 136–137.

Porter, Meredith L., and Beth L. Dennis. "Hyperbilirubinemia in the Term Newborn." *American Family Physician* 65, no. 4 (2002): 599–607.

Read by QxMD. "Effects of Paternal Skin-to-Skin Contact in Newborns and Fathers After Cesarean Delivery." read.qxmd.com/read/30676465/effects-of-paternal-skin-to-skin-contact-in-newborns-and-fathers-after-cesarean-delivery.

Sanberg, Paul R., Dong-Hyuk Park, and Cesar V. Borlongan. "Stem Cell Transplants at Childbirth." *Stem Cell Reviews and Reports* 6 (2010): 27–30.

Schoen, Edgar J., Michael Oehrli, Christopher D. Colby, and Geoffrey Machin. "The Highly Protective Effect of Newborn Circumcision Against Invasive Penile Cancer." *Pediatrics* 105, no. 3 (March 2000): E36. doi.org/10.1542/peds.105.3.e36.

Selander, Jodi, Allison Cantor, Sharon M. Young, and Daniel C. Benyshek. "Human Maternal Placentophagy: A Survey of Self-Reported Motivations and Experiences Associated with Placenta Consumption." *Ecology of Food and Nutrition* 52 , no. 2 (2013): 93–115.

Shankar, K. R., and A. M. Rickwood. "The Incidence of Phimosis in Boys." *BJU International* 84, no. 1 (1999): 101–102. doi.org/10.1046/j.1464-410x.1999.00147.x.

Shearer, M. J. "Vitamin K Metabolism and Nutriture." *Blood Reviews* 6, no. 2 (1992): 92–104. pubmed.ncbi.nlm.nih.gov/1633511/.

Shizhen, Li. *Compendium of Materia Medica: Bencao Gangmu*. Vol. 6. Beijing: Foreign Language Press, 2006, pp. 4182–4186.

Singh-Grewal, Davinder, J. Macdessi, and Jonathan Craig. "Circumcision for the Prevention of Urinary Tract Infection in Boys: A Systematic Review of Randomised Trials and Observational Studies." *Archives of Disease in Childhood* 90, no. 8 (August 2005): 853–858.

Starts Hear. "Hearing Loss Help." www.startshear.org/hearing-loss-help.

Smith, Hazel A., and Genevieve E. Becker. "Early Additional Food and Fluids for Healthy Breastfed Full-Term Infants." *Cochrane Database of Systematic Reviews*, no. 8 (August 30, 2016).

Sorokan, S. Todd, Jane C. Finlay, Ann L. Jefferies, and Canadian Paediatric Society, Fetus and Newborn Committee, Infectious Diseases and Immunization Committee. "Newborn Male Circumcision." *Paediatric Child Health* 20, no. 6 (2015): 311–315. doi.org/10.1093/pch/20.6.311.

UNICEF UK. "Skin-to-Skin Contact." www.unicef.org.uk/babyfriendly/news-and-research/baby-friendly-research/research-supporting-breastfeeding/skin-to-skin-contact/.

Van Hasselt, Peter M., Tom J. de Koning, Nina Kvist, Elsemieke de Vries, Christina Rydahl Lundin, Ruud Berger, Jan L. L. Kempen, Roderick H. J. Houwen, Marianne Hørby Jørgensen, and Henkjan J. Verkade. "Prevention of Vitamin K Deficiency Bleeding in Breastfed Infants: Lessons from the Dutch and Danish Biliary Atresia Registries." *Pediatrics* 121, no. 4 (2008): e857–e863.

Weiss, Helen A., Natasha Larke, Daniel Halperin, and Inon Schenker. "Complications of Circumcision in Male Neonates, Infants and Children: A Systematic Review." *BMC Urology* 10 (2010): 2. www.cdc.gov/mmwr/preview/mmwrht/1471-2490-10-2.

WHO Multicentre Growth Reference Study Group. "WHO Child Growth Standards Based on Length/Height, Weight and Age." *Acta Paediatrica* 450 (suppl, 2006): 76–85.

Williams, Brian G., James O. Lloyd-Smith, Eleanor Gouws, Catherine Hankins, Wayne M. Getz, John Hargrove, Isabelle de Zoysa, Christopher Dye, and Bertran Auvert. "The Potential Impact of Male Circumcision on HIV in Sub-Saharan Africa." *PLoS Medicine* 3, no. 7 (July 2006): e262. doi.org/10.1371/journal.pmed.0030262.

Yao, Alice C., and John Lind. "Effect of Early and Late Cord Clamping on the Systolic Time Intervals of the Newborn Infant." *Acta Paediatrica Scandinavica* 66 (1977): 489–493.

Young, Sharon M., and Daniel C. Benyshek. "In Search of Human Placentophagy: A Cross-Cultural Survey of Human Placenta Consumption, Disposal Practices, and Cultural Beliefs." *Ecology of Food and Nutrition* 49, no. 6 (2010): 467–484. doi.org/10.1080/03670244.2010.524106.

Young, Sharon M., Laura K. Gryder, Winnie B. David, Yuanxin Teng, Shawn Gerstenberger, and Daniel C. Benyshek. "Human Placenta Processed for Encapsulation Contains Modest Concentrations of 14 Trace Minerals and Elements." *Nutrition Research* 36, no. 8 (August 2016): 872–878.

SECTION II: COMING HOME

American Academy of Pediatrics. "American Academy of Pediatrics Issues Clinical Practice Guidelines for Fever in Infants Ages 8 Days–60 Days." Accessed September 12, 2023. www.aap.org/en/news-room/news-releases /aap/2021/american-academy-of-pediatrics-issues-clinical-practice -guidelines-for-fever-in-infants-ages-8-days-60-days.

American Academy of Pediatrics Task Force on Infant Positioning and SIDS. "Positioning and SIDS." *Pediatrics* 89, no. 6 (1992): 1120–1126. publications .aap.org/pediatrics/article-abstract/89/6/1120/57959/Positioning-and-SIDS.

American Academy of Pediatrics Task Force on Infant Sleep Position and Sudden Infant Death Syndrome. "Changing Concepts of Sudden Infant Death Syndrome: Implications for Infant Sleeping Environment and Sleep Position." *Pediatrics* 105, no. 3 (2000): 650–656.

American Pregnancy Association. "Baby Blues." americanpregnancy.org/healthy -pregnancy/first-year-of-life/baby-blues/.

———. "Key Facts About Colic." americanpregnancy.org/healthy-pregnancy /first-year-of-life/colic/.

Anderson, Mark E., Daniel C. Johnson, and Holly A. Batal. "Sudden Infant Death Syndrome and Prenatal Maternal Smoking: Rising Attributed Risk in the Back to Sleep Era." *BMC Medicine* 3, no. 4 (2005).

REFERENCES

Arnett, Megan, and Science Buddies. "Diapers: What Keeps Babies (and Astronauts) from Springing a Leak?" *Scientific American*, August 25, 2016. www.scientificamerican.com/article/diapers-what-keeps-babies-and-astronauts-from-springing-a-leak/.

Banks, J. B., Audra S. Rouster, and J. Chee. "Infantile Colic." *StatPearls*. Treasure Island, FL: StatPearls Publishing, 2023.

Barr, Ronald G. "Colic and Crying Syndromes in Infants." *Pediatrics* 102, no. 5. (1998): 1282–1286.

Bernstein, Aaron S., Emily Oken, Sarah de Ferranti, Jennifer Ann Lowry, Samantha Ahdoot, Carl R. Baum, Aparna Bole, Lori G. Byron, Philip J. Landrigan, Steven M. Marcus, et al. "Fish, Shellfish, and Children's Health: An Assessment of Benefits, Risks, and Sustainability." *Pediatrics* 143, no. 6 (2019). doi.org/10.1542/peds.2019-0999.

Blair, Peter S., Peter J. Fleming, Iain J. Smith, Martin Ward Platt, Jeanine Young, Pam Nadin, P. J. Berry, and Jean Golding. "Babies Sleeping with Parents: Case-Control Study of Factors Influencing the Risk of the Sudden Infant Death Syndrome." *BMJ* 319, no. 7223 (1999): 1457–1461.

Bombard, Jennifer M., Katherine Kortsmit, Lee Warner, Carrie K. Shapiro-Mendoza, Shanna Cox, Charlan D. Kroelinger, Sharyn E. Parks, Deborah L. Dee, Denise V. D'Angelo, Ruben A. Smith, et al. "Vital Signs: Trends and Disparities in Infant Safe Sleep Practices—United States, 2009–2015." *Morbidity and Mortality Weekly Report (MMWR)* 67, no. 1 (2018): 39–46.

Bouillon, Roger, Lieve Verlinden, and Annemieke Verstuyf. "Is Vitamin D2 Really Bioequivalent to Vitamin D3?" *Endocrinology* 157, no. 9 (2016): 3384–3387. doi.org/10.1210/en.2016-1528.

Brazelton, T. B. "Crying in Infancy." *Pediatrics* 29 (1962): 579–588. pubmed.ncbi.nlm.nih.gov/13872677/.

Burger, Joanna. "Fishing, Fish Consumption, and Awareness About Warnings in a University Community in Central New Jersey in 2007, and Comparisons with 2004." *Environmental Research* 108, no. 1 (2008): 107–116.

Canani, Roberto Berni, Pia Cirillo, Paola Roggero, Claudio Romano, Basilio Malamisura, Gianluca Terrin, Annalisa Passariello, Francesco Manguso, Lorenzo Morelli, and Alfredo Guarino. "Therapy with Gastric Acidity Inhibitors Increases the Risk of Acute Gastroenteritis and Community-Acquired Pneumonia in Children." *Pediatrics* 117, no. 5 (2006): e817–e820.

Carpenter, R. G., L. M. Irgens, P. S. Blair, P. D. England, P. Fleming, J. Huber, G. Jorch, and P. Schreuder. "Sudden Unexplained Infant Death in 20 Regions in Europe: Case Control Study." *The Lancet* 363, no. 9404 (2004): 185–191.

Centers for Disease Control and Prevention. "Sudden Unexpected Infant Death and Sudden Infant Death Syndrome: Data and Statistics." www.cdc.gov/sids/data.htm.

Cleveland Clinic. "Postpartum Depression." my.clevelandclinic.org/health/diseases/9312-postpartum-depression.

Clifford, Tammy J., M. Karen Campbell, Kathy N. Speechley, and Fabian Gorodzinsky. "Infant Colic: Empirical Evidence of the Absence of an Association with Source of Early Infant Nutrition." *Archives of Pediatrics & Adolescent Medicine*. 156, no. 11 (2002): 1123–8. doi.org/10.1001/archpedi.156.11.1123.

Corwin, Michael, and Eve Colson. National Infant Sleep Position Study (Version 1). NICHD Data and Specimen Hub. 2016.

Durrant, Louise R., Giselda Bucca, Andrew Hesketh, Carla Möller-Levet, Laura Tripkovic, Huihai Wu, Kathryn H. Hart, John C. Mathers, Ruan M. Elliott, Susan A. Lanham-New, and Colin P. Smith. "Vitamins D_2 and D_3 Have Overlapping but Different Effects on the Human Immune System Revealed Through Analysis of the Blood Transcriptome." *Frontiers in Immunology* 13 (2022): 790444.

Franco, Patricia, Sonia Scaillet, Vanessa Wermenbol, F. Valente, J. Groswasser, and A. Kahn. "The Influence of a Pacifier on Infants' Arousals from Sleep." *Journal of Pediatrics* 136, no. 6 (2000): 775–779.

Guo, Joshua, Z. Goldenberg, Claire Humphrey, Regina El Dib, and Bradley C. Johnston. "Probiotics for the Prevention of Pediatric Antibiotic Associated Diarrhea." *Cochrane Database of Systematic Reviews* 4, no. 4 (April 30, 2019). doi.org/10.1002/14651858.cd004827.pub5.

Hauck, Fern R., John M. D. Thompson, Kawai O. Tanabe, Rachel Y. Moon, and Mechtild M. Vennemann. "Breastfeeding and Reduced Risk of Sudden Infant Death Syndrome: A Meta-Analysis." *Pediatrics* 128, no. 1 (2011): 103–110.

Healthy Children. "All Children Need Vitamin D." Accessed September 12, 2023. www.healthychildren.org/English/healthy-living/nutrition/Pages/vitamin-d-on-the-double.aspx.

———. "Are Some Babies at Higher Risk for SIDS?" www.healthychildren.org/English/tips-tools/ask-the-pediatrician/Pages/are-some-babies-at-higher-risk-for-sids.aspx.

———. "Vitamin D on the Double." Accessed September 12, 2023. www.healthychildren.org/English/healthy-living/nutrition/Pages/vitamin-d-on-the-double.aspx.

Henrick, Bethany M., Lucie Rodriguez, Tadepally Lankshmikanth, Christian Pou, Ewa Henckel, Aron Arzoomand, Axel Olin, Jun Want, Jaromir Mikes, Ziyang Tan, et al. "Bifidobacteria-Mediated Immune System Imprinting Early in Life." *Cell* 184, no. 15 (July 22, 2021): 3884–3898.

Hodgman, Joan E., and Toke Hoppenbrouwers. "Home Monitoring for the Sudden Infant Death Syndrome. The Case Against." *Annals of the New York Academy of Sciences* 533 (1988): 164–175.

Hoffman, Howard J., Marian Willinger, Carol R. Levinson, Christine H. Chong, Yvonne M. Smith, Scott C. Steinschneider, James J. Collins, and Henry F. Krous. "Maternal and Infant Factors Influencing Neonatal Deaths due to Sudden Infant Death Syndrome (SIDS) in the United States: Trends and Disparities." *Journal of Paediatrics and Child Health* 53, no. 2 (2017): 130–135.

Hollis, Bruce W., Carol L. Wagner, Cynthia R. Howard, Myla Ebeling, Judy R. Shary, Pamela G. Smith, Sarah N. Taylor, Kristen Morella, Ruth A. Lawrence, and Thomas C. Hulsey. "Maternal Versus Infant Vitamin D Supplementation During Lactation: A Randomized Controlled Trial." *Pediatrics* 136, no. 4 (2015): 625–634. doi.org/10.1542/peds.2015-1669.

Illueca, Marta, Berhanu Alemayehu, Nze Shoetan, and Huiying Yang. "Proton Pump Inhibitor Prescribing Patterns in Newborns and Infants. " *Journal of Pediatric Pharmacology and Therapeutics* 19, no. 4 (2014): 283–287.

Johnson, Jeremy D., Katherine Cocker, and Elisabeth Chang. "Infantile Colic: Recognition and Treatment." *American Family Physician* 92, no. 7 (2015): 577–582. www.aafp.org/pubs/afp/issues/2015/1001/p577.html

Kim, Seran. "Colic in Babies: Signs, Causes and What to Do" Babylist, January 30, 2023. www.babylist.com/hello-baby/what-is-colic.

Kuppermann, Nathan, James F. Holmes, Peter S. Dayan, John D. Hoyle Jr., Shireen M. Atabaki, Richard Holubkov, Frances M. Nadel, David Monroe, Rachel M. Stanley, Dominic A. Borgialli, et al. "Identification of Children at Very Low Risk of Clinically-Important Brain Injuries After Head Trauma: A Prospective Cohort Study." *The Lancet* 374, no. 9696 (2009): 1160–1170.

Malchodi, Laura, Kari Wagner, Apryl Susi, Gregory Gorman, and Elizabeth Hisle-Gorman. "Early Acid Suppression Therapy Exposure and Fracture in Young Children." *Pediatrics* 144, no. 1 (2019): e20182625.

Malloy, Michael H. "Trends in Postneonatal Aspiration Deaths and Reclassification of Sudden Infant Death Syndrome: Impact of the 'Back to Sleep' Program." *Pediatrics* 109, no. 4 (2002): 661–665.

March of Dimes. "Baby Blues After Pregnancy." www.marchofdimes.org/find-support/topics/postpartum/baby-blues-after-pregnancy.

———. "Postpartum Depression." www.marchofdimes.org/find-support/topics/postpartum/postpartum-depression.

Maski, Kiran P., and Sanjeev V. Kothare. "Sleep Deprivation and Neurobehavioral Functioning in Children." *International Journal of Psychophysiology* 89, no. 2 (2013): 259–264.

MedlinePlus. "Infantile Colic." medlineplus.gov/ency/patientinstructions/000753.htm.

———. "Reflux in Infants." Accessed September 12, 2023. medlineplus.gov/refluxininfants.html.

Mitchell, E. A., and J. M. Thompson. "Co-Sleeping Increases the Risk of SIDS, but Sleeping in the Parents' Bedroom Lowers it." In *Sudden Infant Death Syndrome: New Trends in the Nineties*. Oslo, Norway: Scandinavian University Press, 1995, pp. 266–269.

Monod, Nicole, Perrine Plouin, Bernadette Sternberg, Patricio Peirano, Nicole Pajot, Robert Flores, Susan Linnett, Bernadette Kastler, Cristina Scavone, and Simone Guidasci. "Are Polygraphic and Cardiopneumographic Respiratory Patterns Useful Tools for Predicting the Risk for Sudden Infant Death Syndrome? A 10-Year Study." *Biological Neonate* 50, no. 3 (1986): 147–153.

Moon, Rachel Y., Rebecca F. Carlin, and Ivan Hand. "Sleep-Related Infant Deaths: Updated 2022 Recommendations for Reducing Infant Deaths in the Sleep Environment." American Academy of Pediatrics, Policy Statement. *Pediatrics* 150, no. 1 (2022).

Moskal, Emily. "Infant Gut Microbiome & Breast Milk." *Stanford Medicine*, June 10, 2022. Accessed September 12, 2023. med.stanford.edu/news/all-news/2022/06/infant-gut-microbiome-breast-milk.html.

Mughal, Saba, Yusra Azhar, and Waquar Siddiqui. "Postpartum Depression." *StatPearls*. NCBI Bookshelf, 2022. www.ncbi.nlm.nih.gov/books/NBK519070/.

National Institute of Child Health and Human Development. "Back Sleeping and Reducing the Risk of Sudden Infant Death Syndrome (SIDS)." safetosleep.nichd.nih.gov/research/science/backsleeping#f1.

———. "What Causes SIDS?" safetosleep.nichd.nih.gov/about/causes.

National Institutes of Health. "Combined Prenatal Smoking, Drinking Greatly Increases SIDS Risk." www.nih.gov/news-events/news-releases/combined-prenatal-smoking-drinking-greatly-increases-sids-risk.

National Institutes of Health, Office of Dietary Supplements. "Omega-3 Fatty Acids." Accessed September 12, 2023. ods.od.nih.gov/factsheets/Omega3FattyAcids-HealthProfessional/.

Oddy, Wendy H., Nicholas H. de Klerk, Garth E. Kendall, Seema Mihrshahi, and Jennifer K. Peat. "Ratio of Omega-6 to Omega-3 Fatty Acids and Childhood Asthma." *Journal of Asthma* 41, no. 3 (2004): 319–326. doi.org/10.1081/jas-120026089.

Olm, Matthew R., Dylan Dahan, Matthew M. Carter, Bryan D. Merrill, Feiqiao B. Yu, Sunit Jain, Xiandong Meng, Surya Tripathi, Hannah Wastyk, Norma Neff, et al. "Robust Variation in Infant Gut Microbiome Assembly Across a Spectrum of Lifestyles." *Science* 376, no. 6598 (June 9, 2022): 1220–1223. doi.org/10.1126/science.abj2972.

Osher, Yuly, and Robert H. Belmaker. "Omega-3 Fatty Acids in Depression: A Review of Three Studies." *CNS Neuroscience & Therapeutics* 15, no. 2 (2009): 128–133. doi.org/10.1111/j.1755-5949.2008.00061.x.

Patel, Aakash K., Vamsi Reddy, Karlie R. Shumway, and John F. Araujo. "Physiology, Sleep Stages." *StatPearls* 2022. www.ncbi.nlm.nih.gov/books/NBK526132/.

Poole, S. R. "The Infant with Acute, Unexplained, Excessive Crying." *Pediatrics* 88 (1991): 450–455.

Raiha, Harri, Lehtonen Leo, Korhonen Timo, and Korvenranta Heikki. "Family Life 1 Year After Infantile Colic." *Archives of Pediatrics & Adolescent Medicine* 150 (1996): 1032–1036.

Ramanathan, Rangasamy, Michael J. Corwin, Carl E. Hunt, George Lister, Larry R. Tinsley, Terry Baird, Jean M. Silvestri, David H. Crowell, David Hufford, Richard J. Martin, et al. "Cardiorespiratory Events Recorded on Home Monitors: Comparison of Healthy Infants with Those at Increased Risk for SIDS." *JAMA* 285, no. 17 (2001): 2199–2207.

Rechtman, Lauren R., Jeffrey D. Colvin, Peter S. Blair, and Rachel Y. Moon. "Sofas and Infant Mortality." *Pediatrics* 134, no. 5 (2014): e1293–e1300.

Saghir, Zahid, Javeria N. Syeda, Adnan S. Muhammad, and Tareg H. Balla Abdalla. "The Amygdala, Sleep Debt, Sleep Deprivation, and the Emotion of Anger: A Possible Connection?" *Cureus* 10, no. 7 (2018). doi.org/10.7759/cureus.2912.

Stewart, Dan, and William Benitz. "Umbilical Cord Care in the Newborn Infant." *Pediatrics* 138, no. 3 (2016): e20162149. doi.org/10.1542/peds.2016-2149.

Stewart, Dan, William Benitz, Kristi L. Watterberg, James J. Cummings, William E. Benitz, Eric C. Eichenwald, Brenda B. Poindexter, Dan L. Stewart, Susan W. Aucott, Jay P. Goldsmith, et al. "Umbilical Cord Care in the Newborn Infant." *Pediatrics* 138, no. 3 (2016). doi.org/10.1542/peds.2016-2149.

Stonehouse, Welma. "Does Consumption of LC Omega-3 PUFA Enhance Cognitive Performance in Healthy School-Aged Children and Throughout Adulthood? Evidence from Clinical Trials." *Nutrients* 6, no. 7 (2014): 2730–2758. doi.org/10.3390/nu6072730.

Sung, Valerie, Frank D'Amico, Michael D. Cabana, Kim Chau, Gideon Koren, Francesco Savino, Hania Szajewaska, Girish Desphande, Christophe Dupont, Flavia Indrio, et al. "*Lactobacillus reuteri* to Treat Infant Colic: A Meta-Analysis." *Pediatrics* 141, no. 1 (January 2018): e20171811. doi.org/10.1542/peds.2017-1811.

Swanson, Danielle, Robert Block, and Shaker A. Mousa. "Omega-3 Fatty Acids EPA and DHA: Health Benefits Throughout Life." *Advances in Nutrition* 3, no. 1 (2012): 1–7.

Tablizo, Mary Anne, Penny Jacinto, Dawn Parsley, Maida Lynn Chen, Rangasamy Ramanathan, and Thomas G. Keens. "Supine Sleeping Position Does Not Cause Clinical Aspiration in Neonates in Hospital Newborn Nurseries." *Archives of Pediatrics & Adolescent Medicine* 161, no. 5 (2007): 507–510.

Tappin, David, Russell Ecob, and Hazel Brooke. "Bed Sharing, Room Sharing, and Sudden Infant Death Syndrome in Scotland: A Case-Control Study." *Pediatrics* 147, no. 1 (2005): 32–37.

Terrin, Gianluca, Annalisa Passariello, Mario De Curtis, Francesco Manguso, Gennaro Salvia, Laura Lega, Francesco Messina, Roberto Paludetto, and Roberto Berni Canani. "Ranitidine Is Associated with Infections, Necrotizing Enterocolitis, and Fatal Outcome in Newborns." *Pediatrics* 129, no. 1 (2012): e40–e45. pubmed.ncbi.nlm.nih.gov/22157140/.

Trachtenberg, Felicia L., Elisabeth A. Haas, Hannah C. Kinney, Christina Stanley, and Henry F. Krous. "Risk Factor Changes for Sudden Infant Death Syndrome After Initiation of Back-to-Sleep Campaign." *Pediatrics* 129, no. 4 (2012): 630–638.

Wales, Danielle, Leisa Skinner, and Melanie Hayman. "The Efficacy of Telehealth-Delivered Speech and Language Intervention for Primary School-Age Children: A Systematic Review." *International Journal of Telerehabilitation* 13, no. 1 (2021): 41–60.

Ward, Sally L. Davidson, Thomas G. Keens, Linda S. Chan, Bradley E. Chipps, Stephen H. Carson, Douglas D. Deming, Vijaya Krishna, Hugh M. MacDonald, Gilbert I. Martin, Keith S. Meredith, et al. "Sudden Infant Death Syndrome in Infants Evaluated by Apnea Programs in California." *Pediatrics* 77, no. 4 (1986): 451–458.

Weiss, Peter P., and Reinhold Kerbl. "The Relatively Short Duration That a Child Retains a Pacifier in the Mouth During Sleep: Implications for Sudden Infant Death Syndrome." *European Journal of Pediatrics* 160, no. 1 (2001): 60–70.

Wolf, Elizabeth R., Roy T. Sabo, Martin Lavallee, Evan French, Alan R. Schroeder, Alison N. Huffstetler, Matthew Schefft, and Alex H. Krist. "Overuse of Reflux Medications in Infants." *Pediatrics* 151, no. 3 (2022). publications.aap.org/pediatrics/article/151/3/e2022058330/190640/Overuse-of-Reflux-Medications-in-Infants.

Zermiani, Angela Pierina Dos Reis Buzzo, Ana Luiza Pelissari Peçanha de Paula Soares, Bárbara Leticia da Silva Guedes de Moura, Edson Roberto Arpini Miguel, Luciana Dias Ghiraldi Lopes, Natália de Carvalho Scharf Santana, Thais da Silva Santos, Izabel Galhardo Demarchi, and Jorge Juarez Teixeira. "Evidence of *Lactobacillus reuteri* to Reduce Colic in Breastfed Babies: Systematic Review and Meta-Analysis." *Complementary Therapies in Medicine* 63 (December 2021): 102781.

SECTION III: FROM BABY TO TODDLER

Abrams, Elissa M., and Allan B. Becker. "Food Introduction and Allergy Prevention in Infants." *CMAJ* 187, no. 17 (2015): 1297–1301.

American Academy of Pediatrics. *Caring for Your Baby and Young Child: Birth to Age 5*. 7th ed. New York: Bantam, 2016.

———. "Discipline and Your Child." In *Guidelines for Effective Discipline*. Elk Grove Village, IL: American Academy of Pediatrics, 2016.

REFERENCES

American Speech-Language-Hearing Association. "Early Identification of Speech, Language, Swallowing, and Hearing Disorders." www.asha.org/public/early-identification-of-speech-language-and-hearing-disorders/.

———. "Typical Speech and Language Development." www.asha.org/public/speech/development/chart/.

Andrillon, Thomas, Yuval Nir, Chiara Cirelli, Giulio Tononi, and Itzhak Fried. "Single-Neuron Activity and Eye Movements During Human REM Sleep and Awake Vision." *Nature Communications* 8 (2017): 324.

The Associated Press. "A Missouri School District Reinstated Spanking If Parents Give Their OK." NPR, August 27, 2022. www.npr.org/2022/08/27/1119790279/missouri-school-district-spanking-parents.

Barquet, Nicolau, and Pere Domingo. "Smallpox: The Triumph over the Most Terrible of the Ministers of Death." *Annals of Internal Medicine* 127, no. 8 Pt 1 (1997): 635–642.

Bassil, Kate L., Cathy Vakil, M. Sanborn, Donald C. Cole, Judith Salmon Kaur, and Kathleen J. Kerr. "Cancer Health Effects of Pesticides: Systematic Review." *Canadian Family Physician* 53, no. 10 (October 2007): 1704–1711.

Baumrind, Diana. "Child Care Practices Anteceding Three Patterns of Preschool Behavior." *Genetic Psychology Monographs* 75, no. 1 (1967): 43–88.

———. "Effects of Authoritative Parental Control on Child Behavior." *Child Development* 37, no. 4 (1966): 887–907.

Berk, Laura E., and Adena B. Meyers. "The Role of Make-Believe Play in the Development of Executive Function: Status of Research and Future Directions." *American Journal of Play* 6, no. 1 (2013): 98–110.

Berry, Janet, Mervyn Griffiths, and Carolyn Westcott. "A Double-Blind, Randomized, Controlled Trial of Tongue-Tie Division and Its Immediate Effect on Breastfeeding." *Breastfeeding Medicine* 7, no. 3 (2012): 189–193.

Bjorklund, David F., and Brandi L. Green. "The Adaptive Nature of Cognitive Immaturity." *American Psychologist* 47, no. 1 (1992): 46–54.

Black, Maureen M. "Zinc Deficiency and Child Development." *American Journal of Clinical Nutrition* 68, no. 2 (1998): 464S–469S.

Brown, A. "No Difference in Self-Reported Frequency of Choking Between Infants Introduced to Solid Foods Using a Baby-Led Weaning or Traditional Spoon-Feeding Approach." *Journal of Human Nutrition and Dietetics* 31, no. 4 (August 2018): 496–504.

Brown, Amy, and Michelle Lee. "A Descriptive Study Investigating the Use and Nature of Baby-Led Weaning in a UK Sample of Mothers." *Maternal & Child Nutrition* 7, no. 1 (2011): 34–47.

Burnett, Mark E., and Steven Q. Wang. "Current Sunscreen Controversies: A Critical Review." *Photodermatology, Photoimmunology & Photomedicine* 27, no. 2 (2011): 58–67.

Centers for Disease Control and Prevention. "Breastfeeding and Alcohol." Accessed September 14, 2023. www.cdc.gov/breastfeeding/breastfeeding-special-circumstances/vaccinations-medications-drugs/alcohol.html.

———. "Breastfeeding Report Card." www.cdc.gov/breastfeeding/data/reportcard.htm.

———. "Cronobacter Infection: Technical Information." www.cdc.gov/cronobacter/technical.html#how-common.

———. "Data & Statistics on Autism Spectrum Disorder." www.cdc.gov/ncbddd/autism/data.html.

———. "History of Smallpox." www.cdc.gov/smallpox/history/history.html.

———. "Insect Repellent Use & Safety." www.cdc.gov/niosh/topics/outdoor/mosquito-borne/repellents.html

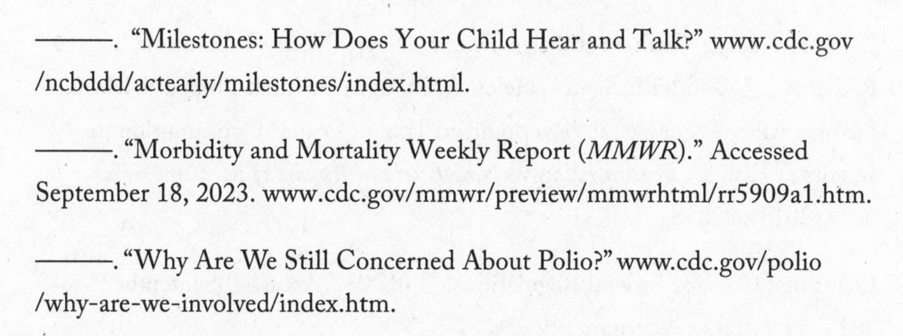

———. "Milestones: How Does Your Child Hear and Talk?" www.cdc.gov/ncbddd/actearly/milestones/index.html.

———. "Morbidity and Mortality Weekly Report (*MMWR*)." Accessed September 18, 2023. www.cdc.gov/mmwr/preview/mmwrhtml/rr5909a1.htm.

———. "Why Are We Still Concerned About Polio?" www.cdc.gov/polio/why-are-we-involved/index.htm.

Chang, Anne-Marie, Daniel Aeschbach, Jeanne F. Duffy, and Charles A. Czeisler. "Evening Use of Light-Emitting eReaders Negatively Affects Sleep, Circadian Timing, and Next-Morning Alertness." *Proceedings of the National Academy of Sciences* 112, no. 4 (2015): 1232–1237.

Choi, Seunghyuk, Dae Ki Hong, Bo Young Choi, and Sang Won Suh. "Zinc in the Brain: Friend or Foe?" *International Journal of Molecular Sciences* 21, no. 23 (2020): 8941.

Christakis, Dimitri A. "Interactive Media Use at Younger than the Age of 2 Years: Time to Rethink the American Academy of Pediatrics guideline?" *JAMA Pediatrics* 168, no. 5 (2014): 399–400.

Committee on Practice and Ambulatory Medicine, Committee on Infectious Diseases, Committee on State Government Affairs, Council on School Health, Section on Administration and Practice Management. "Medical Versus Nonmedical Immunization Exemptions for Child Care and School Attendance." *Pediatrics* 138, no. 3 (2016): e20162145.

DiMaggio, Dina M., Amanda Cox, and Anthony F. Porto. "Updates in Infant Nutrition." *Pediatrics in Review* 38, no. 10 (2017): 449–462.

Downs, Craig A., Esti Kramarsky-Winter, Roee Segal, John Fauth, Sean Knutson, Omri Bronstein, Frederic R. Ciner, Rina Jeger, Yona Lichtenfeld, Cheryl M. Woodley, et al. "Toxicopathological Effects of the Sunscreen UV Filter, Oxybenzone (Benzophenone-3), on Coral Planulae and Cultured Primary Cells." *Archives of Environmental Contamination and Toxicology* 70, no. 2 (2016): 265–288.

Du Toit, George, Graham Roberts, Peter H. Sayre, Henry T. Bahnson, Suzana Radulovic, Alexandra F. Santos, Helen A. Brough, Deborah Phippard, Monica Basting, Mary Feeney, et al. "Randomized Trial of Peanut Consumption in Infants at Risk for Peanut Allergy." *New England Journal of Medicine* 372, no. 9 (2015): 803–813.

Electronic Code of Federal Regulations. "Title 21." Accessed September 18, 2023. www.ecfr.gov/current/title-21.

Endocrine Society. "Plastics, EDCs & Health: Authoritative Guide." December 10, 2020. www.endocrine.org/topics/edc/plastics-edcs-and-health.

Fangupo, Louise J., Anne-Louise M. Heath, Sheila M. Williams, Liz W. Erickson Williams, Brittany J. Morison, Elizabeth A. Fleming, Barry J. Taylor, Benjamin J. Wheeler, and Rachael W. Taylor. "A Baby-Led Approach to Eating Solids and Risk of Choking." *Pediatrics* 138, no. 4 (2016): e20160772.

Fidler Mis, Nataša, Christian Braegger, Jiri Bronsky, Cristina Campoy, Magnus Domellöf, Nicholas D. Embleton, Iva Hojsak, Jessie Hulst, Flavia Indrio, Alexandre Lapillonne, et al. "Sugar in Infants, Children and Adolescents: A Position Paper of the European Society for Paediatric Gastroenterology, Hepatology and Nutrition Committee on Nutrition." *Journal of Pediatric Gastroenterology and Nutrition* 65, no. 6 (December 2017): 681–696.

Finkelhor, David, Heather Turner, Brittany Kaye Wormuth, Jennifer Vanderminden, and Sherry Hamby. "Corporal Punishment: Current Rates from a National Survey." *Journal of Child and Family Studies* 28 (2019): 1991–1997. doi.org/10.1007/s10826-019-01426-4.

Fukunaka, Ayako, and Yoshio Fujitani. "Role of Zinc Homeostasis in the Pathogenesis of Diabetes and Obesity." *International Journal of Molecular Sciences* 19, no. 2 (2018): 476.

Gershoff, Elizabeth T., and Andrew Grogan-Kaylor. "Spanking and Child Outcomes: Old Controversies and New Meta-Analyses." *Journal of Family Psychology* 30, no. 4 (2016): 453–469.

Ginsburg, Kenneth R. "The Importance of Play in Promoting Healthy Child Development and Maintaining Strong Parent-Child Bonds." *Pediatrics* 119, no. 1 (2007): 182–191.

Goldman, Armond S. "Evolution of Immune Functions of the Mammary Gland and Protection of the Infant." *Breastfeeding Medicine* 7, no. 3 (2012): 132–142.

Gracián-Alcaide, Carlos, Jose A. Maldonado-Lobón, Elisabeth Ortiz-Tikkakoski, Alejandro Gómez-Vilchez, Juristo Fonollá, Jose L. López-Larramendi, Mónica Olivares, and Ruth Blanco-Rojo. "Effects of a Combination of Elderberry and Reishi Extracts on the Duration and Severity of Respiratory Tract Infections in Elderly Subjects: A Randomized Controlled Trial." *Applied Sciences* 10, no. 22 (2020): 8259.

Grandjean, Philippe, and Philip J. Landrigan. "Neurobehavioural Effects of Developmental Toxicity." *The Lancet Neurology*. 30, no. 3 (2014): 330–338.

Greer, Frank R., Scott H. Sicherer, A. Wesley Burks, Robert D. Baker, Jatinder J. S. Bhatia, Stephen Robert Daniels, Marcie B. Schneider, Janet Silverstein, and Dan W. Thomas. "Effects of Early Nutritional Interventions on the Development of Atopic Disease in Infants and Children: The Role of Maternal Dietary Restriction, Breastfeeding, Timing of Introduction of Complementary Foods, and Hydrolyzed Formulas." *Pediatrics* 121, no. 1 (2008): 183–191.

Haastrup, Maija Bruun, Anton Pottegård, and Per Damkier. "Alcohol and Breastfeeding." *Basic Clinical Pharmacology Toxicology* 114, no. 2 (February 2014): 168–173. doi.org/10.1111/bcpt.12149.

Hafez, Lamia M., Hebatallah Mohammed Aboudeya, Noura A. Matar, Ashraf S. El-Sebeay, Azhar Mohamed Nomair, Shaymaa Ali El-Hamshary, Hanan Mohamed Nomeir, and Fawziya A. R. Ibrahim. "Ameliorative Effects of Zinc

Supplementation on Cognitive Function and Hippocampal Leptin Signaling Pathway in Obese Male and Female Rats." *Scientific Reports* 13, no. 5072 (2023).

Hilton, Courtney B., Cody J. Moser, Mila Bertolo, Harry Lee-Rubin, Dorsa Amir, Constance M. Bainbridge, Jan Simson, Dean Knox, Luke Glowacki, Elias Alemu, et al. "Acoustic Regularities in Infant-Directed Speech and Song Across Cultures." *Natural Human Behaviour* 6 (2022): 1545–1556.

Holick, Michael F. "Vitamin D Deficiency." *New England Journal of Medicine* 357, no. 3 (2007): 266–281.

Hopkins, Donald R. *Princes and Peasants: Smallpox in History*. Chicago: University of Chicago Press, 1983.

Hultman, Christina M., Sven Sandin, Stephen Zvi Levine, Paul Lichtenstein, and Abraham Reichenberg. "Advancing Paternal Age and Risk of Autism: New Evidence from a Population-Based Study and a Meta-Analysis of Epidemiological Studies." *Epidemiology* 16, no. 12 (2011): 1203–12.

Imdad, Aamer, and Zulfiqar A. Bhutta. "Effect of Preventive Zinc Supplementation on Linear Growth in Children Under 5 Years of Age in Developing Countries: A Meta-analysis of Studies for Input to the Lives Saved Tool." *BMC Public Health* 11, no. S3 (2011): S22.

Iweala, Onyinye I., Shailesh K. Choudhary, and Scott P. Commins. "Food Allergy." *Current Gastroenterology Reports* 20, no. 5 (2018): 17.

Koren, Gideon. "Drinking Alcohol While Breastfeeding. Will It Harm My Baby?" *Canadian Family Physician* 48 (2002): 39–41.

Krause, M., A. Klit, M. Blomberg Jensen, T. Søeborg, H. Frederiksen, M. Schlumpf, W. Lichtensteiger, N. E. Skakkebaek, and K. T. Drzewiecki. "Sunscreens: Are They Beneficial for Health? An Overview of Endocrine Disrupting Properties of UV-Filters." *International Journal of Andrology* 35, no. 3 (2012): 424–436.

REFERENCES

Kuhl, Patricia K. "Early Language Learning and Literacy: Neuroscience Implications for Education." *Mind, Brain, and Education* 5, no. 3 (2011): 128–142. doi.org/10.1111/j.1751-228X.2011.01121.x.

Lieberthal, Allan S., Aaron E. Carroll, Tasnee Chonmaitree, Theodore G. Ganiats, Alejandro Hoberman, Mary Anne Jackson, Mark D. Joffe, Donald T. Miller, Richard M. Rosenfeld, Xavier D. Sevilla, et al. "The Diagnosis and Management of Acute Otitis Media." 131, no. 3 (2013): e964–e999. doi.org/10.1542/peds. 2012-3488.

Logan, Jessica A. R., Laura M. Justice, Melike Yumuş, and Leydi Johana Chaparro-Moreno. "When Children Are Not Read To at Home: The Million Word Gap." *Journal of Developmental and Behavioral Pediatrics* 40, no. 5 (2019): 383–386. doi.org/10.1097/DBP.0000000000000657.

Lyons, Albert S., and R. Joseph Petrucelli II. *Medicine: An Illustrated History.* New York: Harry N. Abrams, 1997.

Maccoby, Eleanor E., and John A. Martin. "Socialization in the Context of the Family: Parent-Child Interaction." *Handbook of Child Psychology: Vol. 4. Socialization, Personality, and Social Development*, edited by Paul H. Mussen, 1–101. New York: Wiley, 1983.

Mason, Sherri A, Victoria G. Welch, and Joseph Neratko. "Synthetic Polymer Contamination in Bottled Water." *Frontiers in Chemistry* 11, no. 6 (September 11, 2018): 407. doi.org/10.3389/fchem.2018.00407.

McLeod, Sharynne, and Kathryn Crowe. "Children's Consonant Acquisition in 27 Languages: A Cross-Linguistic Review." *American Journal of Speech-Language Pathology* 27, no. 4 (2018): 1546–1571. doi.org/10.1044/2018_AJSLP-17-0100.

Meek, Joan Younger, Lawrence Noble, and Section on Breastfeeding. "Policy Statement: Breastfeeding and the Use of Human Milk." *Pediatrics* 150, no. 1 (July 2022): e2022057988.

Mehus, Christopher J., and Megan E. Patrick. "Prevalence of Spanking in US National Samples of 35-Year-Old Parents from 1993 to 2017." *JAMA Pediatrics* 175, no. 1 (2021): 92–94. doi.org/10.1001/jamapediatrics.2020.2197.

Mindell, Jodi A., Brett Kuhn, Daniel S. Lewin, Lisa J. Meltzer, and Avi Sadeh. "Behavioral Treatment of Bedtime Problems and Night Wakings in Infants and Young Children." *Sleep* 29, no. 10 (2006): 1263–1276.

Mohammad, Mohammad K., Zhanxiang Zhou, Matthew Cave, Ashutosh Barve, and Craig J. McClain. "Zinc and Liver Disease." *Nutrition in Clinical Practice* 27, no. 1 (2012): 8–20. doi.org/10.1177/0884533611433534. Erratum in: *Nutrition in Clinical Practice* 27, no. 2 (April 2012): 305.

Montgomery-Downs, Hawley E., Heather M. Clawges, and Eleanor E. Santy. "Infant Feeding Methods and Maternal Sleep and Daytime Functioning." *Pediatrics* 126, no. 6 (2010): e1562–e1568.

Morison, Brittany J., Rachael W. Taylor, Jillian J. Haszard, Claire J. Schramm, Liz Williams Erickson, Louise J. Fangupo, Elizabeth A. Fleming, Ashley Luciano, and Anne-Louise M. Heath. "How Different Are Baby-Led Weaning and Conventional Complementary Feeding? A Cross-Sectional Study of Infants Aged 6–8 Months." *BMJ Open* 6, no. 5 (2016): e010665.

Muraro, A., S. Halken, S. H. Arshad, K. Beyer, A. E. Dubois, G. Du Toit, P. A. Eigenmann, K. E. C. Grimshaw, A. Hoest, G. Lack, L. O'Mahony, et al. "EAACI Food Allergy and Anaphylaxis Guidelines. Primary Prevention of Food Allergy." *Allergy* 69, no. 5 (2014): 590–601.

Murray, Robert D. "Savoring Sweet: Sugars in Infant and Toddler Feeding." *Annals of Nutrition and Metabolism* 70, no. S3 (2017): S38–S46.

National Institute on Deafness and Other Communication Disorders. "Speech and Language." www.nidcd.nih.gov/health/speech-and-language.

Ostrov, Jamie M., Kathleen E. Woods, Elizabeth A. Jansen, Juan F. Casas, and Nicki R. Crick. "An Observational Study of Delivered and Received Aggression, Gender, and Social-Psychological Adjustment in Preschool: 'This White Crayon Doesn't Work . . . '." *Early Childhood Research Quarterly* 19, no. 2 (2004): 355–371.

Owens, Judith A., Anthony Spirito, and Melissa McGuinn. "The Children's Sleep Habits Questionnaire (CSHQ): Psychometric Properties of a Survey Instrument for School-Aged Children." *Sleep* 23, no. 8 (December 15, 2000): 1043–1051.

Paruthi, Shalini, Lee J. Brooks, Carolyn D'Ambrosio, Wendy A. Hall, Suresh Kotagal, Robin M. Lloyd, Beth A. Malow, Kiran Maski, Cynthia Nichols, Stuart F. Quan, et al. "Recommended Amount of Sleep for Pediatric Populations: A Consensus Statement of the American Academy of Sleep Medicine." *Journal of Clinical Sleep Medicine* 12, no. 6 (2016): 785–786.

Paul, Rhea. *Language Disorders from Infancy Through Adolescence: Assessment & Intervention*. St. Louis, MO: Mosby, 2006.

Perkin, Michael R., Kirsty Logan, Anna Tseng, Bunmi Raji, Salma Ayis, Janet Peacock, Helen Brough, Tom Marrs, Suzana Radulovic, Joanna Craven, et al. "Randomized Trial of Introduction of Allergenic Foods in Breast-Fed Infants." *New England Journal of Medicine* 374, no. 18 (2016): 1733–1743.

Pfeiffer, Carl C., and Eric R. Braverman. "Zinc, the Brain, and Behavior." *Biological Psychology* 17, no. 4 (1982): 513–532.

Potegal, Michael, and Richard J. Davidson. "Temper Tantrums in Young Children: 1. Behavioral Composition." *Journal of Developmental and Behavioral Pediatrics* 24, no. 3 (2003): 140–147.

Prasad, Ananda S. "Impact of the Discovery of Human Zinc Deficiency on Health." *Journal of Trace Elements in Medicine and Biology* 28, no. 4 (2014): 357–363.

Radesky, Jenny S., Jayna Schumacher, and Barry Zuckerman. "Mobile and Interactive Media Use by Young Children: The Good, the Bad, and the Unknown." *Pediatrics* 135, no. 1 (2015): 1–3.

Ramírez-Esparza, Nairán, Adrián García-Sierra, and Patricia K. Kuhl. "Look Who's Talking: Speech Style and Social Context in Language Input to Infants Are Linked to Concurrent and Future Speech Development." *Developmental Science*. 17, no. 6 (2014): 880–891.

Repacholi, Betty M., Andrew N. Meltzoff, Theresa M. Hennings, and Ashley L. Ruba. "Transfer of Social Learning Across Contexts: Exploring Infants' Attribution of Trait-Like Emotions to Adults." *Infancy* 21, no. 6 (2016): 785–806.

Richardson, Alexandra J. "Omega-3 Fatty Acids in ADHD and Related Neuro-developmental Disorders." *International Review of Psychiatry* 18, no. 2 (2006): 155–72.

Richardson, Alexandra J., Jennifer R. Burton, Richard P. Sewell, Thees F. Spreckelsen, and Paul Montgomery. "Docosahexaenoic Acid for Reading, Cognition and Behavior in Children Aged 7–9 Years: A Randomized, Controlled Trial (the DOLAB Study)." *PloS One* 7, no. 9 (2012): e43909.

Riedel, Stefan. "Edward Jenner and the History of Smallpox and Vaccination." *Proceedings of the Baylor University Medical Center* 18, no. 1 (2005): 21–25.

Riley, Claudette. "Missouri School District Reinstates Spanking as Punishment: 'We've Had People Actually Thank Us.'" *Springfield News-Leader*, August 23, 2022. www.news-leader.com/story/news/education/2022/08/23/missouri-school-district-reinstates-spanking-corporal-punishment-cassville/7872893001/.

Rose, V., D. Trembath, D. Keen, and J. Paynter. "The Proportion of Minimally Verbal Children with Autism Spectrum Disorder in a Community-Based Early Intervention Programme." *Journal of Intellectual Disability Research* 60, no. 5 (2016): 464–477. doi.org/10.1111/jir.12284.

Sabbatani, Sergio, and Sirio Fiorino. "La peste antonina e il declino dell'Impero Romano. Ruolo della guerra partica e della guerra marcomannica tra il 164 e il 182 d.C. nella diffusione del contagio [The Antonine Plague and the Decline of the Roman Empire]." *Infezioni in Medicina* 17, no. 4 (2009): 261–275.

Sanborn, M., Kathleen J. Kerr, L. H. Sanin, Donald C. Cole, Kate L. Bassil, and Cathy Vakil. "Non-cancer Health Effects of Pesticides." *Canadian Family Physician* 53, no. 10 (October 2007): 1712–1720.

Sandin, Sven, Paul Lichtenstein, Ralf Kuja-Halkola, Christina Hultman, Henrik Larsson, and Abraham Reichenberg. "The Heritability of Autism Spectrum Disorder." *JAMA* 318, no. 12 (2017): 1182–84.

Sandstead, Harold H. "Nutrition and Brain Function: Trace Elements." *Nutrition Reviews* 44 (Suppl, 1986): S37–S41. doi.org/10.1111/j.1753-4887.1986.tb07676.

Sherman, Amanda L., Julia Anderson, Colin D. Rudolf, and Lynn S. Walker. "Lactose-Free Milk or Soy-Based Formulas Do Not Improve Caregivers' Distress or Perceptions of Difficult Infant Behavior." *AAP Grand Rounds* 34, no. 5 (2015): 49.

Sicherer, Scott H., and Hugh A. Sampson. "Food Allergy: A Review and Update on Epidemiology, Pathogenesis, Diagnosis, Prevention, and Management." *Journal of Allergy and Clinical Immunology* 141, no. 1 (2018): 41–58.

Stoody, Eve E., Joanne M. Spahn, and Kellie O. Casavale. "The Pregnancy and Birth to 24 Months Project: A Series of Systematic Reviews on Diet and Health." *American Journal of Clinical Nutrition* 109, no. S7 (2019): 685S–697S.

Sudakin, Daniel L., and Wade R. Trevathan. "DEET: A Review and Update of Safety and Risk in the General Population." *Journal of Toxicology: Clinical Toxicology* 41, no. 6 (2003): 831–839.

Tarczoń, Izabela, Ewa Cichocka-Jarosz, Anna Knapp, and Przemko Kwinta. "The 2020 Update on Anaphylaxis in Paediatric Population." *Advances in Dermatology and Allergology* 39, no. 1 (2022): 13–19. Published online February 6, 2021. doi.org/10.5114/ada.2021.103327.

Telemo, Esbjörn, and Lars A. Hanson. "Antibodies in Milk." *Journal of Mammary Gland Biology and Neoplasia* 1 (1996): 243–249.

Thèves, Catherine, Eric Crubézy, and Philippe Biagini. "History of Smallpox and Its Spread in Human Populations." *Microbiology Spectrum* 4, no. 4 (2016).

Timby, Niklas, Magnus Domellöf, Bo Lönnerdal, and Olle Hernell. "Supplementation of Infant Formula with Bovine Milk Fat Globule Membranes." *Advances in Nutrition* 8, no. 2 (2017): 351–355.

Togias, Alkis, Susan F. Cooper, Maria L. Acebal, Amal Assa'ad, James R. Baker, Lisa A. Beck, Julie Block, Carol Byrd-Bredbenner, Edmond S. Chan, Lawrence F. Eichenfield, et al. "Addendum Guidelines for the Prevention of Peanut Allergy in the United States: Report of the National Institute of Allergy and Infectious Diseases—Sponsored Expert Panel." *Journal of Allergy and Clinical Immunology* 139, no. 1 (2017): 29–44.

Townsend, Ellen, and Nicola J. Pitchford. "Baby Knows Best? The Impact of Weaning Style on Food Preferences and Body Mass Index in Early Childhood in a Case-Controlled Sample." *BMJ Open* 2, no. 1 (2012): e000298.

US Department of Agriculture, Food Safety and Inspection Service. "Food Product Dating." www.fsis.usda.gov/food-safety/safe-food-handling-and-preparation/food-safety-basics/food-product-dating.

US Department of Agriculture and US Department of Health and Human Services. Dietary Guidelines for Americans. Accessed September 18, 2023. www.dietaryguidelines.gov/.

US Food and Drug Administration. "Questions & Answers for Consumers Concerning Infant Formula." Accessed September 18, 2023. www.fda.gov/food/people-risk-foodborne-illness/questions-answers-consumers-concerning-infant-formula.

———. "Regulations and Information for the Manufacture and Distribution of Infant Formula." Accessed September 18, 2023. www.fda.gov/food/infant-formula-guidance-documents-regulatory-information/regulations-and-information-manufacture-and-distribution-infant-formula.

———. "Title 21—Food and Drugs, Chapter I, Subchapter B, Part 107, Subpart B—Labeling, § 107.100. Infant Formula; Nutrient Requirements; Nutrient Specification; Label Statements." Accessed September 18, 2023. www.accessdata.fda.gov/scripts/cdrh/cfdocs/cfcfr/CFRSearch.cfm?fr=107.100.

Wieland, L. Susan, Vanessa Piechotta, Termeh Feinberg, Emilie Ludeman, Brian Hutton, Salmaan Kanji, Dugald Seely, and Chantelle Garritty. "Elderberry for Prevention and Treatment of Viral Respiratory Illnesses: A Systematic Review." *BMC Complementary Medicine and Therapies* 21, no. 1 (2021): 112.

Woolf, Alan. "Well Water Safety & Testing: AAP Policy Explained." HealthyChildren.org, February 20, 2023. www.healthychildren.org/English/safety-prevention/all-around/Pages/Where-We-Stand-Testing-of-Well-Water.aspx.

World Health Organization. "History of Polio Vaccination." www.who.int/news-room/spotlight/history-of-vaccination/history-of-polio-vaccination.

———. "Smallpox." www.who.int/health-topics/smallpox#tab=tab_1.

Wright, Charlotte M., Kirsty Cameron, Maria Tsiaka, and Kathryn N. Parkinson. "Is Baby-Led Weaning Feasible? When Do Babies First Reach Out For and Eat Finger Foods?" *Maternal & Child Nutrition* 7, no. 1 (2011): 27–33.

Zablotsky, Benjamin, Lindsay I. Black, and Lara J. Akinbami. "NCHS Data Brief, no. 459: Diagnosed Allergic Conditions in Children Aged 0–17 Years: United States, 2021." National Center for Health Statistics, 2023.

Zero to Three. "Tuning in: Parents of Young Children Speak Up About What They Think, Know and Need." Washington, DC: Zero to Three, 2016.

Acknowledgments

I wish to dedicate this book to my incredible wife, Sarah, and our wonderful son, Eli. I am also profoundly grateful to my parents, Ian and Hedy, to my siblings, Erica and Steven, and to my family-in-law, Irene, Alex, and Brandon.

Special appreciation goes to Libby Edelson, whose instrumental role in transferring the contents of my mind to the page cannot be overstated. Without you, this book would not exist. Your leadership, guidance, and wisdom have breathed life into these pages.

Thank you to my amazing agent, Coleen O'Shea, my fantastic editor, Jessica Firger, and the amazing team at Union Square & Co.

Most important, this book is a dedication to all the extraordinary parents out there. It is a tribute to you, for your children, both present and future. Allow me to articulate what your children are unable to express at this time.

Parents, I salute your remarkable strength, love, and sacrifice. From sleepless nights and endless cuddles to ceaseless support and guidance, you are the real-life superheroes who mold our existence.

Your unwavering devotion has reared us. Thank you for your limitless patience and unconditional love. Your presence in our lives is a daily treasure.

Your nurturing nature and unending affection lay down a bedrock of love that will guide us throughout our lives.

To the working parents, balancing their careers and family lives, your resilience and determination are awe-inspiring. You demonstrate that it's possible to chase our dreams while also nurturing our families, and for that, we salute you.

To the single parents, you exemplify strength and resilience. Your capacity to manage everything single-handedly is nothing short of miraculous. Your love knows no bounds, and your children are lucky to have you as their compass.

To the grandmothers and grandfathers, thank you for imparting your wisdom, love, and traditions through generations. Your loving embrace and soothing words provide a unique sense of security and belonging.

To the stepparents, adoptive parents, and all those who step into parental roles, opening their hearts and homes, you are a lighthouse of love and acceptance. You fill our lives with joy immeasurable, patching gaps and building bridges.

This book is a celebration of, and a dedication to, not just our own parents, but also the parent figures who have touched our lives in countless ways. If circumstances permit, take a moment to call your parents and express your love to them.

Index

INDEX

INDEX

INDEX

About the Author

Joel "Gator" Warsh aka @DrJoelGator of the popular parenting Instagram page is a board-certified pediatrician in Los Angeles, California, who specializes in parenting, wellness, and integrative medicine. He grew up in Toronto, Canada, and completed degrees in kinesiology, psychology, and epidemiology, before earning his medical degree from Thomas Jefferson Medical College.

He completed his pediatric medicine training at one of the top five residency programs in the country, Children's Hospital of Los Angeles (CHLA) and then worked in private practice in Beverly Hills before founding his current practice, Integrative Pediatrics and Medicine Studio City, in 2018.

Dr. Gator has published research in premier peer-reviewed journals on topics including childhood injuries, obesity, and physical activity.

He has been featured in numerous documentaries, films, summits, podcasts, and articles by CBS, Fox, NBC, the *Washington Post*, and many others.

He is also the founder of the parenting masterclass series Raising Amazing, which can be found at RaisingAmazingPlus.com. He is also a consultant for high-profile brands in the health and wellness space.